THE STRENGTH TRAINING WORKOUTS FOR SENIORS 60+ BIBLE

[7 in 1]

The Most Complete Guide of 200+ Simple

Exercises that Elderly of Any Level

Can Do Step by Step at Home

Dorian Ritter

CONTENTS

INTRODUCTION

Aging is just a natural evolution of the human body, it is inevitable, and we cannot slow it down. However, we can listen to the body's changing needs, adapt to a new lifestyle, make better choices, and exercise well to keep the bones, muscles, and mind strong and flexible.

Stiff muscles, cramps, fractures, bad posture, and the fear of falling are some of the most common worries of seniors over 60, and to a greater extent, their apprehensions are not wrong. And for the same reasons, most seniors avoid doing exercises regularly. However, studies show that careful, regular, and light exercise for at least 10-20 minutes a day helps muscles regain their strength and flexibility, which can prevent stiffness and cramps. It is good for physical health, provides mental strength, and enhances cognitive abilities. So, it's a win-win for all.

However, after a certain age, our bones and muscles need extra care, so every exercise must be carried out with safety precautions in a controlled manner. There are various exercises you can try as a senior, and this 7-in-1 exercises for seniors' package has compiled various exercise methods that you can benefit from. You can find them all, from stretching to resistance exercises, home workouts, and core strength exercises.

What Comes with Aging?

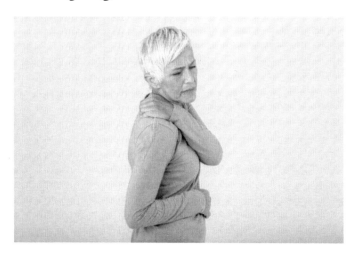

Questions about aging may arise, such as: why our bodies age and how old someone can get. However, getting older is more complicated than simply counting the years you've lived. Our bodies are intricate machines with a vast array of traits and capabilities. Over time, it is typical for our cells and tissue to sustain damage or make errors. In our earlier years, these changes didn't pose an issue because many of them could be easily repaired, or our bodies have the necessary reserves to compensate for them. But as we age, our capacity to repair this harm declines. Thus, it starts to accumulate and results in aging symptoms.

What Happens to Your Body When You Age?

It is believed that your inherited genes, or the DNA in your cells, play a role in determining how old you become. Some individuals might only begin to deteriorate later in life and live longer. However, other elements also have a favorable effect. These include maintaining a healthy lifestyle with frequent exercise, wholesome eating, emotional stability, and a strong social network.

If the injured cells do not recover or die, the organs cannot function as well as they previously did. Over time, several organs also lose bulk (become smaller or "thin out"). However, this shrinkage of reserves is not apparent for a long time because our organs contain enormous reserves to handle the increased load when necessary. The classic aging symptoms start to show only until the reserves have significantly diminished.

However, these aging symptoms aren't health issues, and you may usually delay them for a long time; you can perform workouts to strengthen your muscles, for instance, if they start to weaken. Sports and exercise are thought to be healthy for you, for example, to maintain the health of your other organs and your cardiovascular system (heart and blood vessels).

The Typical Signs of Aging

From the outside, it is possible to see several aging symptoms: your skin develops wrinkles and age spots, and your hair begins to grey. As we become older, our bodies become less able to hold fluid, which causes, for example, our spinal discs to shrink and lose their suppleness. As a result, as humans age, they become smaller. This alteration typically occurs in the body's organs and tissues over a long time without being immediately apparent. Some people don't show them until they are extreme stress or elderly age. Others experience this sooner.

As we age, messages take longer to travel along our nerves, and our brains are less able to interpret information than they once were. This makes it more difficult to recall new information and respond promptly. Our sensory systems also deteriorate over time; for example, it's common to experience age-related nearsightedness in your mid-forties and hearing issues as you get older. Over time, you may also lose the ability to taste and smell certain things.

What Does Growing Older Mean?

Growing older entails a variety of experiences and changes, both psychologically and physically. Our body and mind adjust to outside forces at all life stages, including aging. This can gradually and unconsciously occur over time, for instance, throughout your job or family life. Or it might occur more overtly and on purpose, like while practicing for an athletic event or recovering from a terrible illness.

For as long as they live, people are constantly changing. Loss, limits, and the difficulty of continually adjusting to new conditions can all be symptoms of aging. However, because aging often occurs slowly, this adaptation proceeds over time. You go through many changes with your family and friends since they age alongside you. When things go tough, staying physically active and utilizing your life experience and insight will help you overcome many of the obstacles you encounter.

Contentment and happiness are as important in later years as in early ones. Numerous elderly persons enjoy retirement, free from many pre-existing expectations and limitations. Others are content to have more time for themselves, their loved ones, and their friends, while some search for new tasks. Staying active for as long as possible is physically and mentally crucial.

Why is It Necessary to Exercise?

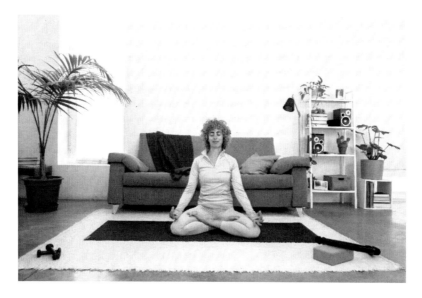

Exercise is unquestionably the best prescription for maintaining health and reducing aging throughout a lifetime. Researchers at the University of Birmingham and King's College London compared the muscles and immune systems of older persons who had consistently exercised throughout their lives to those of adults of comparable age and younger adults who had not routinely exercised. They discovered that people who exercised regularly fought against the effects of aging by possessing the immunity and muscle mass of someone significantly younger. Aging alone does not result in a reduction of immunological defense. Instead, the cause is a lack of activity.

We now have solid evidence that encouraging people to commit to physical activity throughout their lives is a potential solution to the problem since we are living longer but not healthier. Regular exercise should start by late middle age (before age 65) and be done four to five times a week to reap the greatest benefits.

A few aging-related changes begin as early as the third decade of life. For instance, after age 25 to 30, the average man's maximum attainable heart rate and peak blood pump capacity fall by roughly one beat per minute and ten percent, respectively. Because of this, a healthy 25-year-old heart can pump 212 quarts of blood in a minute, but a heart that is 65 years old or older can only pump 112 quarts, and a heart that is 80 years old or older can only pump approximately a quart in a minute. With simple daily tasks, this decreased aerobic capacity might result in exhaustion and shortness of breath.

A man's blood vessels start to tighten in middle age, and his blood pressure usually rises. Even though there are fewer oxygen-carrying red blood cells in his circulation, the blood changes, becoming thicker and stickier and more difficult to circulate through the body.

Most Americans start gaining weight in their middle years, adding 3–4 pounds annually. However, that extra weight is all fat because men begin to lose muscle in their 40s. This additional fat makes it more likely for **LDL** ("bad") cholesterol to increase and **HDL** ("good") cholesterol to decrease. Additionally, it explains why type 2 diabetes, distressingly prevalent in older people, rises by around 6 points every ten years in blood sugar levels.

Mindset and Motivation

You've heard it repeatedly: exercising and being physically active are good for you, and you should attempt to fit them into your daily schedule. Numerous studies have shown that exercise provides important health advantages, which increase with age. By improving your physical and mental health, regular exercise, and physical activity, seniors can help you maintain your independence as you age. The five advantages of exercise for elders and aging adults are listed below:

Prevent Disease

Regular physical activity can prevent several common diseases, such as diabetes and

heart disease. Generally speaking, exercise improves immune function, which is important for seniors whose immune systems are typically weaker. Simple workouts like walking can aid in managing ailments that can be avoided.

Improved Mental Health

There are several benefits of exercise for mental wellness. Endorphins, the "feel good" hormone that lowers stress and instills feelings of happiness and contentment, are released during exercise. Exercise has been linked to improved sleep, which is important for older people with insomnia and irregular sleep patterns.

Decreased Risks of Falls

Older people are more likely to fall, which could be disastrous for maintaining independence. Exercise reduces the likelihood of falls by improving strength, flexibility, and coordination while improving balance and balance. Anything that can be done to prevent falls in the first place is crucial because senior fall recovery durations are much longer.

Social Engagement

Whether you join a walking club, participate in group fitness classes, or drop by a gardening club, exercising can be a fun social activity. For elderly people to feel a sense of purpose and avoid loneliness or despair, maintaining strong social connections is essential. The most important step is choosing an enjoyable hobby so that working out never feels like a job.

Improved Cognitive Function

The development of motor skills and regular exercise is beneficial for cognitive function. Numerous studies show active persons have a lower risk of dementia regardless of when they first adopt an activity habit.

Safety Precautions

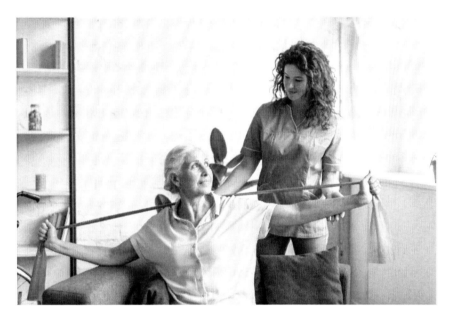

A healthy lifestyle and exercise go hand in hand. Even as you become older, this is true. Unfortunately, the hazards of exercise rise with age, but it shouldn't stop you from exercising. The benefits usually outweigh the drawbacks. You may exercise as safely as you did younger with a few simple steps.

Be Reasonable

Your ultimate fitness objective can be to be in shape enough to compete on a specific date or to complete ten laps of the pool. In any way, make this objective attainable. Remember that most of us will never achieve supermodel or sportsman status. Consider what you are capable of.

Goals Should Be Written Down

Be specific; avoid making your final objective a blanket declaration like, "I want to reduce weight." create a metric for it. How many pounds of weight do you aim to lose precisely?

Select a goal that has value and significance for you, not anyone else. For instance, if your partner wants you to reduce weight, but you are content with how you look, committing to a lifestyle you don't want could be challenging.

Exercise Can Be Risky Business

As you age, your body changes; you lose bone density and muscle mass, and your balance and coordination suffer. Seniors are more susceptible to fractures and falls due to these changes. The heart also changes. According to the national academy of sports medicine, diseases like arteriosclerosis and hypertension become more common as people age. Due to these modifications, seniors should seek a doctor's approval before beginning an exercise program, particularly if they were previously inactive or had a chronic illness.

Wear Appropriate Footwear and Clothing

According to the national institute on aging, think of your shoes as your feet's safety gear. Adapt your footwear to the activity you've chosen. If you stroll, for instance, wear walking shoes instead of tennis shoes. Pick comfortable shoes with supportive heels and non-skid soles that are well-fitted and comfortable. Another precaution is ensuring your shoes are in good condition; the tread should be substantial and unworn. According to the national institute on aging, you shouldn't have fatigue in your feet after wearing them. Your clothes protect you from injury, just like your shoes do. Your clothing should be loose and comfortable enough to allow for easy mobility.

Know When to Stop

Never should exercising be painful. Stop working out as soon as you feel any pressure or pain in your chest or elsewhere and see a doctor. Be alert for any symptoms of weakness, breathlessness, or dizziness. Be mindful of your heart. Call your doctor immediately if your heart skips beats or beats too quickly.

Get Moving Safely

To prevent dehydration, consume 6 to 8 ounces of water. Additionally, avoid working out when it's too hot. The national academy of sports medicine advises older persons to engage in moderate-intensity exercises three to five days per week. Perform these exercises for 30 to 60 minutes. This can be divided into easier, shorter sessions that last 10 minutes each. Make sure to start every workout with at least five minutes of gentle movement. Start your treadmill walk, for instance, at a slow pace. Choose cardio machines with reliable handrail support and an emergency stop button if you do use them.

Stay Hydrated

It's estimated that moderate chronic dehydration affects 25% of senior persons. Eight to ten glasses of water daily are advised to maintain optimal hydration. Older persons have a higher risk of dehydration because:

- **Simply due to old age:** As we get older, we feel less thirst, which lessens our urge to drink.
- **Fear of incontinence:** People who are afraid of being incontinent may refrain from drinking since they usually associate doing so with going to the restroom.
- **Reduced mobility:** This can prevent people from getting themselves a drink because they can't always get to the bathroom, but it can also make them stop drinking.

Pay Attention to Nutrition

A healthy, balanced diet can give your body the resources to function properly.

Our bodies require nutrients from food to function and flourish. They contain water, vitamins, minerals, proteins, lipids, and carbohydrates. Having a healthy diet is crucial at any age. It provides you with energy and can aid with weight management.

Additionally, it might aid in preventing various conditions like osteoporosis, high blood pressure, heart disease, type 2 diabetes, and particular malignancies. However, as you get older, your life and body change, so do the things you need to keep healthy. For instance, even if your caloric needs are lower, you still need to consume enough nutrients. Some elderly people require additional protein. If you want to age well, you should:

- Consume meals that are high in nutrients but low in calories, such as
- Veggies and fruits (choose different types with bright colors)
- Oatmeal, whole-wheat bread, and brown rice are examples of whole grains.
- milk and cheese that are fat-free or low-fat, as well as soy or rice milk with calcium and vitamin D supplements
- Eggs, poultry, lean meats, seafood, nuts, seeds, and beans
- Beware of empty calories. These include foods high in calories but low in nourishment, such as crisps, candy, baked products, soda, and alcohol

Choose foods that are low in fat and cholesterol. Saturated and trans fats should be avoided in particular. Animal fats are often where saturated fats come from. Stick margarine and vegetable shortening contain trans fats, which are processed fats. Some fast-food establishments may use them in their pre-made fried dishes and baked items.

BOOK 1:
HOME WORKOUT FOR SENIORS

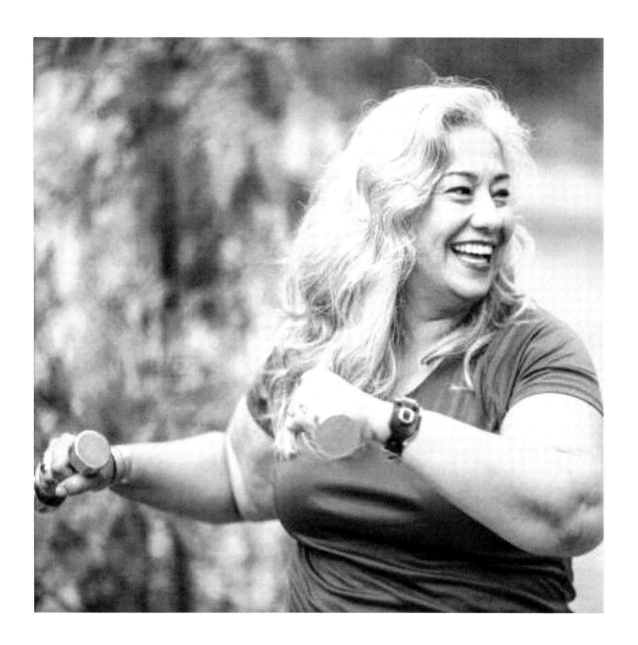

CHAPTER 1: GETTING STARTED WITH TRAINING

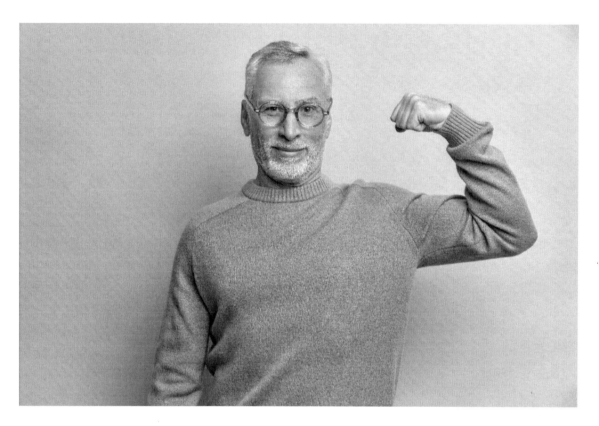

The physical activity guidelines for Americans suggest that you engage in at least 150 minutes (2 ½ hours) of moderate-intensity activity each week, such as brisk walking or quick dancing. The ideal activity level is at least three days a week, but any activity is preferable to inactivity. For instance, attempt balancing training along with cardio and muscle-building exercises.

Exercise and physical activity are amazing for your physical and mental well-being and enhance mobility as you age. This chapter will teach you about some considerations before beginning a fitness regimen.

When starting a physical activity routine, the secret to success and safety is growing gently from your fitness level. Injury from over-exercising can result in giving up. The ideal strategy is continuous advancement. To be cautious and lower your chance of harm:

- Start slowly with low-intensity workouts in your exercise regimen.

- Exercise should be warmed up before and then cooled down.
- Be aware of your surroundings when working out outdoors.
- Even if you don't feel thirsty, hydrate yourself with water before, during, and after your workout.
- Put on the proper footwear and workout attire for your activities.
- Talk to your healthcare physician about your exercise and physical activity plan if you have any particular health issues.

It's also important to note your improvement and progress as the days go by. To begin, record your starting point in your activity log. For a few days, record your usual activity levels; try to pick a couple of weekdays and one weekend day.

Don't forget to assess your fitness level for each of the four workout categories: strength, balance, flexibility, and endurance. Even if you are in good shape to run, you won't profit as much if you don't stretch after your workout.

As you continue your workouts, note your results so that you can monitor your improvement. Take notes on how you feel during the test tasks. If the workouts are challenging, start easy and gradually increase. If they were simple, you would know that you were more physically fit. You can set higher goals for yourself and push yourself.

How Should Workouts Be Structured?

What then makes up a balanced exercise regimen? The following exercises are recommended for everyone to include in their weekly regimens. Seventy-five minutes per week of severe aerobic exercise or 150 minutes of moderate aerobic exercise (for instance, 30 minutes spread out over five days). At least 48 hours must pass between strength training sessions, which should be performed twice or more each week.

If this sounds overwhelming, remember that workouts may be broken into smaller, more doable segments. For example, you can reach your daily goal by taking three 10-minute walks. Additionally, each activity should begin with a brief warm-up and end with a brief cool-down.

To loosen up your muscles and increase the flow of oxygen-rich blood, your warm-up should include light movement like marching in place. After five to ten minutes of reduced activity and intensity, cool down by stretching to help prevent stiffness. Continue reading for additional information on each element of a balanced exercise routine in greater detail and suggestions for various workouts and activities to get you started.

If you're an older adult planning to start an exercise program, your ideal week would include 150 minutes of moderate endurance exercise. To increase strength, flexibility, and balance, spend some time walking, swimming, or cycling daily.

For Americans 65 and older in generally good health, the Centers for Disease Control and Prevention advises this period. Even though this seems like a lot, the good news is that you can split it up into 10- or 15-minute workout sessions twice or more daily. You may perform dozens of workouts to increase your strength without ever setting foot inside a gym. For those just starting, here are a few pointers.

Warm Up

As you warm up, your muscles receive nutrient-rich, oxygenated blood as your heart rate and breathing rate increase. All major muscle groups should be worked during a five to ten-minute warm-up. Start softly, then ramp up the speed for optimal results.

Numerous warm-up programs emphasize cardio and range-of-motion exercises, like lunges and jumping jacks. If you'd like, you can warm up more quickly by dancing to a few songs or walking in place while gently swinging your arms.

Workout Boosters

Balance, core strengthening, and resistance band exercises must be a part of your fitness routine because unintentional falls are a major cause of injuries for many older persons. Walking on uneven surfaces without losing balance is simpler by engaging in balance exercises like the ones mentioned below and sports like tai chi or yoga. You can practice your balance while waiting in line at the bank or the grocery store. You can do these exercises daily, several times daily.

Cool Down

After your workout, it's recommended that you spend five to ten minutes gradually cooling down. This reduces cramping and dizziness as your breathing and heart rate gradually slow.

Stretching exercises are key to a healthy cool-down since they expand your range of motion, relax your body's tight muscles, and alleviate stiff ones. Maintain each stretch for 10 to 30 seconds to benefit from these workouts. The more time you can spend holding a stretch, the more flexible you'll get. Similar to the warm-up, it is best to transition swiftly and without hesitating between each stretch.

Exercises Seniors Can Perform At Home

Seniors should try to work out each week. They can locate a fitness plan that works for them, regardless of whether they are still active or have restricted mobility. Here are five activities that senior citizens can perform at home.

Light Weight Training

Seniors who lift light weights can maintain their bone density and increase muscle mass without overtaxing their muscles. Seniors can perform workouts like shoulder presses and arm lifts using 2-pound weights. They can utilize household items like food or water cans if they don't have weights.

Aerobics

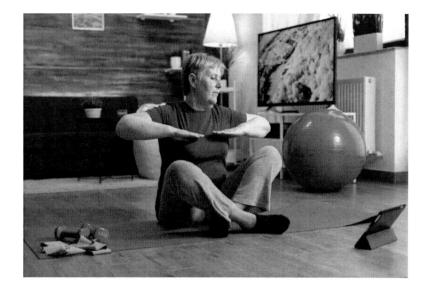

Seniors can perform aerobic exercises without having a gym membership. They can utilize an exercise DVD if they want to stick to a schedule. Many of these DVDs are created especially for seniors. Traditional aerobic exercises like jumping jacks and knee lifts can be performed in 5-minute intervals by older persons who prefer to work alone. Exercises that get the heart beating and improve cardiovascular health are essential.

Yoga

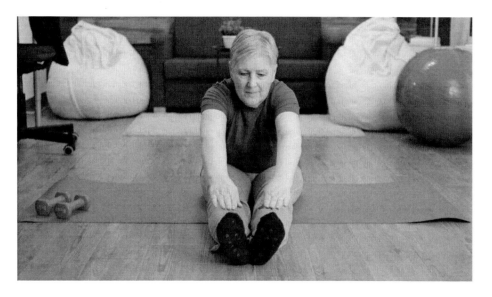

Seniors usually experience joint inflexibility as they age. Yoga is one of the greatest forms of exercise for seniors to maintain flexibility because it emphasizes balance, strength, and strength. Seniors can perform traditional yoga poses, including warrior, seated forward bend, and downward facing dog. Chair yoga is an option for older persons with restricted movement.

Strength Training

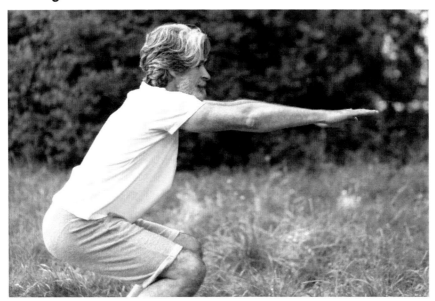

Strength training is a crucial component of any workout program for seniors. Squats train the muscles across the lower body and are one of the best exercises for strengthening the legs.

Begin by standing with your toes pointed forward to execute this exercise. To build muscle in the calves and quads, flex your knees until you are nearly seated and repeat this exercise.

Seniors who require assistance balancing can grab onto a chair. Paying attention to the lower body is important since strong legs can reduce the risk of falls and slips that cause injury.

Walking

Seniors can go for walks without ever leaving the house. They can put on their pedometers, play music, and go for a brisk walk around the house. Seniors should strive to pump their arms and elevate their knees with each step to get the most out of this workout.

How Much Should You Do?

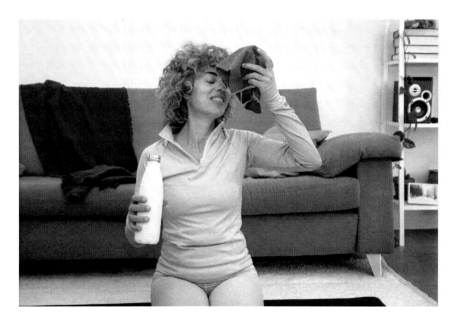

On the major muscle groups (legs, hips, back, chest, abdomen, shoulders, and arms), strengthening exercises should be done twice or more a week, with a minimum of 48 hours in between sessions. While other studies indicate that two or three sets would be preferable, one set per session is effective. Eight to twelve times for each exercise (reps). Your body requires at least 48 hours to recover and repair between strength training sessions to gain muscle mass and strength.

Give Muscles Time Off

Tiny tears in muscle tissue are brought on by demanding exercise, such as strength training. These tears are beneficial, not harmful; when they knit together, the muscles get stronger. Always give muscles at least 48 hours to heal in between exercises. Therefore, if you perform a challenging full-body strength training on Monday, wait until Wednesday before repeating it. The days in between your strength training sessions are ok for aerobic exercise. However, if you're conducting a partial-body strength program, you might exercise your upper body on Monday, lower body on Tuesday, upper body on Wednesday, lower body on Thursday, etc. You may also exercise your cardiovascular system as often as you can.

How to Get Started

Put form first, not size. Correctly position your body and move easily during each exercise. Injuries may result from improper form. Many experts advise beginners undertaking a strength training routine to start with no or extraordinarily little weight. While isolating a muscle group, focus on gradual, fluid lifts and equally controlled descents. You can isolate muscles by keeping your body in a particular position and deliberately tightening and releasing the targeted muscles.

Tempo

Instead of negating the momentum-driven strength increases, tempo aids control. For instance, lift a dumbbell while counting to four, hold it for two seconds, and then drop it to the starting position while counting to four.

Breathe

While exercising, blood pressure rises; however, if you hold your breath while doing weight training, blood pressure rises even more. Exhale as you raise, press, or pull; inhale as you release to prevent sharp rises. Count your tempo out loud to ensure you're not holding your breath. When speaking, you cannot hold your breath.

Keep Pushing Your Muscles

Depending on the exercise, a different weight is appropriate. Select a weight that allows you to retain proper technique while tiring the targeted muscle by the last two repetitions (reps). Pick a smaller weight if you can't complete the required repetitions. You should push your muscles again by adding weight (approximately 1- 2 pounds for arms, 2-5 pounds for legs), using a harder resistance band, or stopping when it feels too simple, and you could keep completing reps. You can also increase the number of reps you do in your workout (up to three sets) or the number of days you work out each week. If you increase the weight, keep in mind that the targeted muscles should feel fatigued by the last two reps and that you should be able to complete the minimum number of repetitions with the proper technique.

Benefits of Training at Home

Seniors can exercise at home in addition to the gym to increase their stability and balance. Our sense of stability declines as we age, so we must be careful to ensure that everything we do is joyful. Exercise enhances the body's cardiovascular system, which might help with balance and postural sway. Regular exercise improves an aged person's stability and balance, lowering their chance of tripping or falling.

There are several benefits to working out at home. Whether they lift weights, work on their cardiovascular system, or engage in other forms of exercise like yoga, seniors can improve their quality of life by being active as they age.

Seniors who stay active and regularly engage in physical activity can experience better health and well-being than they have in years. Regular physical activity can help them feel happier and have a more positive attitude toward life as they age. They will feel more content and enjoy themselves for the remainder of their golden years. The benefits of exercising at home for seniors outweigh the negative psychological and physical effects by a wide margin. It is a great idea for many seniors to try since it has many benefits for them. Exercise regularly benefits the heart, body, and mind.

CHAPTER 2: CREATING A TRAINING ROUTINE

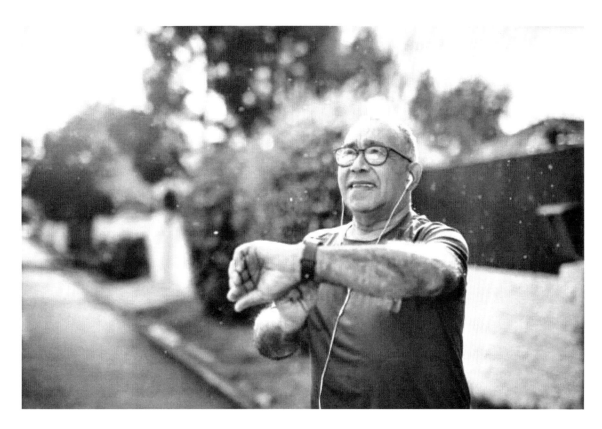

Let's face it; workout equipment is costly. The best ones are priceless and produce amazing results quickly, but hiring a committed trainer is still out of reach for most individuals. That doesn't mean you shouldn't benefit from a smart, well-designed program. You can think like a trainer and create a workout plan that produces the desired outcomes (without spending thousands of dollars at the gym). Continue reading to learn more about creating your workout plan like a pro.

What to Consider when Creating Your Training Routine

The six elements you should consider when creating your plan are listed below.

Consistency

The most important aspect of training consistently is receiving results. You must usually exercise over a long period. Making a program that will keep you in the game should therefore be your priority. However, even the best exercise program is meaningless if you don't follow it. Being sidelined is a definite way to fall short of your objectives, whether due to a lack of development, loss of motivation, or a chronic injury.

Choose whether you'll work out or relax each day by writing the days of the week on a piece of paper. To start, schedule five days of exercise each week and two days of rest. This is more than sufficient for most people to achieve good results. Remember that not every workout day will consist of extreme mileage or tough training; some days may merely feature recuperation or accessory work.

Decide which days you'll train and which days you'll rest for the time being. Choose the five days a week you will engage in some form of exercise. Set a time in your calendar to perform that training at that particular time of day. Commit to completing that training no matter what, keeping in mind that maintaining consistency is key to developing a successful program.

Active Restoration

You've scheduled two days of rest and five days of exercise. Next, choose two days for active recovery: one day for exercise and one day for rest.

Your more severe training should be recovered from with the aid of active recoveries, such as:

- A long walk
- Yoga (at light intensity)
- Foam rolling and myofascial release

You want to stay moving, increase your range of motion, repair your muscles, and preserve an active habit. You can investigate each of the above-mentioned recovery activities on your own (or, even better, try them all and see which ones you enjoy).

A prolonged walk warms up your muscles and joints while also reducing tension. It eases aches and pains from earlier workouts, and when done with gentle stretching, it keeps your range of motion intact (your ability to move fully around any given joint). Similarly, swimming and yoga (done properly and lightly) strengthen your body's dynamic capabilities while keeping you active and having fun.

If your body requires it, you can complete your daily exercise obligation with a simple movement or a workout at a leisurely pace. There's no need to challenge yourself every day.

Variety

We don't want to do too many workouts with the same structure. Usually, changing rep schemes, times, mileage, loads, and activities are required. The best method to cause physical harm and mental exhaustion is to do the same thing every day. Repeating the same movements over and over will wear out your muscles and joints, and eventually, you'll break because the repeated tension will be too much for you to handle. We should choose various activities for each workout day to address our athletic inadequacies while enhancing our strengths.

Challenge

Your workouts need to get harder over time to see consistent improvement. To raise

the relative intensity of your exercises as you go, you must increase the load, speed of completion, volume, or all three. Failure to do this will eventually result in plateauing.

Do Not Complicate Matters

Instead, you should progressively increase the level of challenge while continuing to ensure that you are healing properly from prior workouts. The biggest problem for trainers everywhere is finding the right balance between introducing challenges quickly enough to bring about change without resulting in injury or missing training days.

Before trying to add more difficulty, you should practice for four to six weeks at any particular level and pay attention to your body. You probably scaled the challenge too quickly if you aren't recovering from your workouts well enough to attack the following workout with intensity and attention.

Record Keeping

You must maintain records if you want to follow your program intelligently. You should keep objective and subjective records by noting times, loads, distance, etc. (recording how your body feels, mental state, and recovery level). These records will enable you to see what's working and what isn't, providing information on how to change the program for the following cycle.

Warming Up

Warming up before the exercise is as crucial as learning the right posture for the exercises. It prepares your muscles and bones for the exercises and prevents potential cramps and damage to the body. It has several other benefits as well.

- **Improved Blood Flow:** By warming up for at least 10 minutes with low-intensity activity, you can raise blood volume, reach your skeletal muscles, and expand your blood capillaries. Increased blood flow is one of the most effective ways to ready your muscles for a workout because it transports the oxygen your muscles require to function.

- **Improved Oxygen Efficiency:** When you warm up with exercise, your blood releases oxygen more quickly and at a higher temperature. Your muscles need more oxygen while you exercise; thus, it's important to boost the oxygen's availability through a warm-up activity.

- **Faster Muscle Contraction/Relaxation:** Getting warm through exercise increases body temperature, which enhances nerve conduction and muscle metabolism. The outcome? Your muscles will work more quickly and effectively.

- **Injury Prevention:** By warming up, you can avoid getting hurt. Warming up helps to loosen your joints and boosts blood flow to your muscles, making it less likely for your muscles to rip, tear, or twist during exercise. Additionally, stretching aids in the preparation of your muscles for the upcoming exercise.

- **Mental Preparation:** As you go through the warming process, your mind will start paying more attention to your body and physical activity. Your training session will continue with this concentration, which will aid in developing your technique, coordination, and skill.

Cooling Down

Cooling down activities are carried out after the workout or any particular set of exercises which is important because of the following reasons:

- **Recovery:** Lactic acid accumulates in your system after a vigorous workout, and it takes the body some time to get rid of it. Stretching and other cooling-down exercises can assist in the release and removal of lactic acid, hastening your body's post-workout recovery.

- **Reducing DOMS (Delayed Onset Muscle Soreness):** While some degree of muscle soreness is following normal exercise, many DOMS are extremely uncomfortable and can discourage you from working again. Cycling at a moderate intensity after strength training reduced DOMS. It keeps you more comfortable and enables your body to recover before your next session by reducing excessive muscular soreness after exercise.

Duration and Schedule of Workout

If you're over 50 and recently decided to exercise more, there's a good chance you're thinking a lot. Like, how usually should you perspire? Which workouts should you put first? There are several things to consider, but you may experience additional pains and aches while recuperating. The optimum time of day for you to exercise is something you might not be considering, though.

Although exercise is generally regarded as healthy at any time, the truth is that when you exercise is also significant. According to the prevailing research, there is at least one time of day you would be prudent to avoid.

Don't Work Out 3 Hours Before Bed

Although it may seem enticing to end your day with a workout, studies have shown that doing so within three hours of bed adversely disturbs sleep patterns. The physiological stimulation of working out is the exact opposite of what we want to do as the day ends. In other words, exercise signals our bodies to wake up, which may let you toss and turn till the wee hours of the morning.

A late-night workout may be a waste of time, given how crucial it is for everyone to get a good night's sleep after an intense workout. We exercise for various reasons, including cardiovascular health, lean muscle mass gain, endurance improvement, and more.

Further studies, such as this analysis of 23 earlier studies published in Sports Medicine, have revealed that while evening exercise, in general, may improve sleep, a strenuous workout an hour before bed can make it harder to fall asleep, shorten the amount of time spent sleeping, and reduce the efficiency of sleep in general.

Workout in the Morning

For various reasons, choosing to work out in the morning is preferable. We are all aware that cognitive deterioration usually occurs as we age. Fortunately, studies in the British Journal of

Sports Medicine suggest that early morning exercise can enhance cognition and mental clarity in older persons. Exercise between 8 and 10 a.m. has been found to reduce prostate cancer risk in men and breast cancer in women. According to researchers, this may be because morning activity protects circadian rhythms. Exercise at night can interfere with the body's production of melatonin, the hormone produced when it's time to sleep, which also helps slow cancer growth.

Circadian disturbance, or the misalignment of environmental cues like light and food intake, is one potential risk factor for cancer. Regular physical activity has long been known to lower one's risk of developing cancer. The morning hours are when physical activity may have the greatest protective benefit.

Late Afternoon

Suppose you're just not a morning person; maybe about working out later in the day. Flexibility and strength are often at their peak in the late afternoon. Perceived exertion is at its lowest in the late afternoon, making it possible to increase a workout's intensity without feeling unduly strenuous.

Once more, experts postulate that these findings are connected to humans' intrinsic biological clocks. After waking up each morning, your body temperature progressively increases throughout the day, peaking in the late afternoon.

How to Create Your Personalized Routine

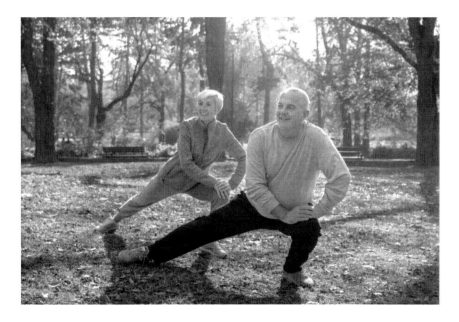

Starting a workout routine is one of the greatest things you can do for your well-being. Exercise can assist you in losing weight, improving your balance and coordination, lowering your risk of developing chronic diseases, and even improving your sleep patterns and self-esteem.

After a certain age, you don't feel as enthuse to exercise as before, and it's fine. You don't have to be too excited about it; you just need the will and intent to stay fit and start somewhere you feel comfortable. You must enjoy your exercises without any pressure on the mind and engage in physical activity with a positive outlook.

Assess Your Abilities

You must first evaluate your skills. Each customized fitness plan begins by considering your present skills. The following three inquiries can help you evaluate your skills.

- What is your body composition?
- What are your movement abilities?
- What is your current level of fitness?

Let's examine each one in more detail and see how it will impact your training schedule.

What is Your Body Composition?

Before beginning your exercise program, I advise you to assess your present body composition. Setting objectives and keeping track of progress can be facilitated by considering your present composition.

Take a picture of yourself or obtain a body analysis so you have something to refer to if your exercise objectives are based on body composition.

What are Your Movement Abilities?

Consider the last time you exercised in a gym. Which movements were easy for you and difficult or even painful? You should keep track of your responses because you'll need them later to choose specific activities. Has your movement been evaluated by a qualified fitness coach for the greatest outcomes?

Answering these questions will help you follow the routine best suited for you. Someone who hasn't been working out for years cannot start by picking up weights and doing heavy strenuous exercises.

What is Your Current Level of Fitness?

You must find the right difficulty level to get as much out of your exercise program. You don't want something that is overly simple or difficult. Your body will be challenged enough during the ideal amount of exercise to maintain consistency.

So, recall the many exercises you've done in the past. What was too difficult, and what was too simple? Note down your response because it will determine the length and nature of your weight-training and cardio exercises.

Assess Your Resources

Take an inventory of your resources for the final component of your assessment. How usually can you exercise each week? How long can you exercise each day? Which exercise tools are available to you? What is your budget for food? You must be aware of your resources. They will directly affect your unique workout schedule.

Define Your Goals

It's time to specify your goals now that you know your starting point. Asking yourself why you want to exercise is a good place to start. Don't settle for the obvious solution after that. Look more closely at your underlying motivations. For instance, why is it vital to you if your objective is to reduce weight? Is it for your family to set an example? Or is it realizing your entire human potential? Whatever it may be, recognizing your genuine reason will make it simpler for you to follow your customized exercise schedule.

Make a smart goal next. This objective is time-based, specific, measurable, achievable, and relevant. An example of gaining muscle would be: "I want to add two pounds of muscle mass in the next two months." I wish to lose 3 pounds of body fat in two months, for instance, if you want to reduce weight. These objectives meet the criteria for smart goals since they are time-based, relevant, precise (several pounds), measurable (pounds can be measured), and realistic (it isn't a lofty aim) (includes a duration of time).

We advise beginning with more manageable goals centered on consistency if you are new to working out. For instance, exercising for 30 minutes three times per week for a month. These more manageable objectives will help you gain confidence as you accomplish them.

Two Types of Workout Plans

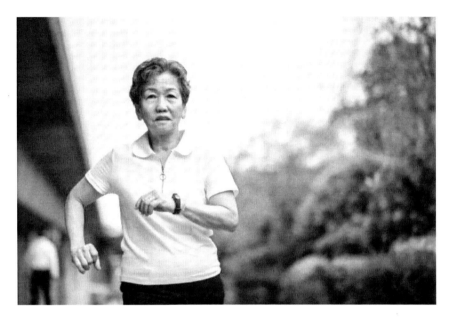

We'll go over how to make two customized exercise schedules: one for beginners and one for more seasoned exercisers. Start with the basic program if you are unsure of where you fall. Even experts will notice improvements.

The Beginner Weekly Training Split

Start by working out four to five times a week. Work out with weights for the entire body on two to three of those days. Do sustained cardio workouts on the other days. These days could involve going to the gym, but they could also involve outdoor sports, walks, hikes, and biking. Throughout the week, alternate between resistance and aerobic exercise.

Advanced Training Split

You probably work out four to six days a week if you are advanced. You can lift weights on two to four of those days. Separate those workout days into days for the upper and lower bodies. Do sustainable aerobic exercises on the other days, and on your off-training days, stroll to stay active.

How to Choose the Right Exercises

Now that you have the weekly split, let's plan out the workouts for each day. Squat, bend, lunge, push, pull, and core movements are all your weight training activities in a gym. Train 5-6 of these patterns each time you work out if you're a beginner.

The advantages of full-body exercises are discussed here. If you are more experienced, separate these movement patterns into workouts for the upper body (push, pull, and core and lower body (squat, bend, lunge, and core).

Choose Rep Ranges, Sets, and Rest Time

When selecting rep ranges for beginners, we like any number between 8 and 15 reps. This is the optimal rep range for increasing muscle endurance and motor control. For novices, 2-4 sets are usually used. To build strength, endurance, and eventually maximal contractions, you can execute fewer repetitions at heavier loads as you improve your training. And lastly, remember to take time to relax. Even though it's common to perform workouts back-to-back for maximal intensity, resting in between sets is crucial. You can perform the same activity at the same intensity after a short rest period.

Quality Over Quantity

The purpose of weight training is to develop movement patterns and build muscle tension. You must keep this in mind and place more emphasis on movement quality than quantity if you want to achieve the finest outcomes. Poorly executed and tense repetitions will promote undesirable tendencies and be unsuccessful. Better than 100 terrible reps are 20 extremely terrific ones.

Create a Cardio Workout Plan

Cardio exercises are aerobic exercises that can be practiced for a long time. Numerous health advantages of cardio include accelerated healing and increased immunological and cognitive function.

Select a form of exercise to construct a cardio workout. We enjoy running, hiking, riding, and rowing. Next, select a timeframe or distance and travel at a speed permitting you to complete the task quickly. Begin by finishing the workout for the allotted time or distance. Then gradually, start extending the time or distance. Your cardio progression will be sustained if you progressively boost the intensity of your exercises over time, which is crucial for building your aerobic system.

How to Deal with Discomfort

Stop exercising altogether if you experience: pain, discomfort, nausea, lightheadedness, dizziness, fainting, chest pain, irregular heartbeat, shortness of breath, or chilly hands. The greatest method to prevent damage is to pay attention to your body. Limit your workouts to 5-10 minutes and instead work out more usually if you consistently feel pain after 15 minutes of activity, for instance.

Avoid using an injured body part in any activity. Exercise your lower body while your upper body recovers if you have an injury and vice versa. After an injury has healed, resume exercise gradually with lesser weights and less resistance.

Get flexible, warm up, and cool down. Warm up with walking for a few minutes, arms swinging, and shoulder rolls, then do some mild stretches (avoid deep stretches when your muscles are cold). After your exercise session—cardiovascular, weight training, or flexibility—cool down with more light movement and deeper stretching. Obtain enough liquids. When your body is well hydrated, it operates at its optimum. Dress appropriately, wearing supportive shoes and loose-fitting, comfortable clothing.

BOOK 2:
STRETCHING EXERCISES
FOR SENIORS

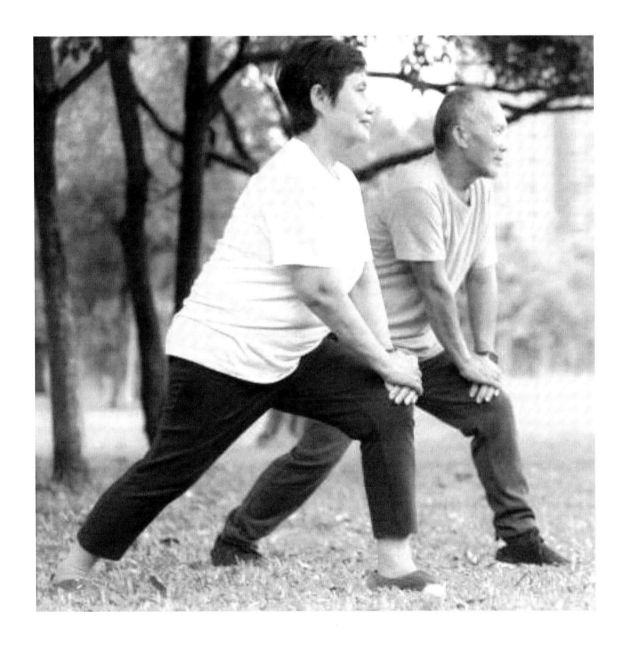

CHAPTER 1: STRETCHING

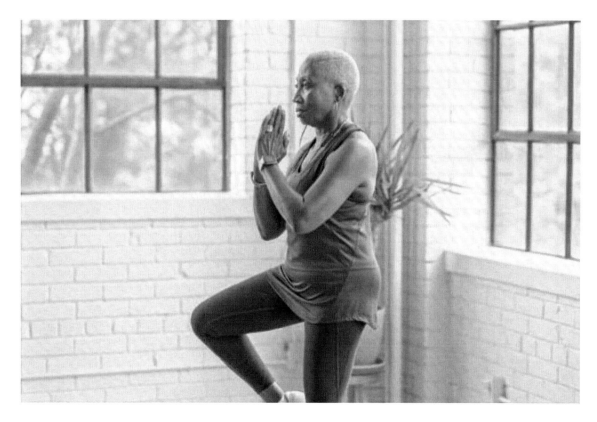

You might have noticed that you're not quite as adaptable as you once were. Daily activities, such as bending over or getting up off the floor, can be harder to complete or stretch far behind or above your head. Or perhaps you have just noticed that your joints aren't moving or straightening out like they used to.

Our bodies will age; it is unavoidable.

Reduced flexibility comes with aging, especially if we overlook what it takes to stay flexible and move well. For older persons, movement, stretching, and exercise are crucial for maintaining their health. But to keep in shape as you age, you don't have to run marathons or bench press like a bodybuilder. Regular exercise and dynamic stretches will help you maintain your fitness level while enhancing your joint and muscle health in addition to a nutritious diet. See your doctor before beginning a new stretching regimen to lessen your risk of injury.

Two distinct kinds of stretches should be recognized: First is static stretching. These often entail contracting specific muscles and holding the stretch for a few seconds. However, this strain won't benefit your muscles if you haven't warmed up. Save the static stretches for your cooldown after your workout. The second is stretching movements which are beneficial to perform as part of your warm-up before a workout. Dynamic stretches involve various actions to stimulate your joints and muscles. It can entail imitating your movements from the sport or activity you're warming up for, but less vigorously.

Benefits of Stretching

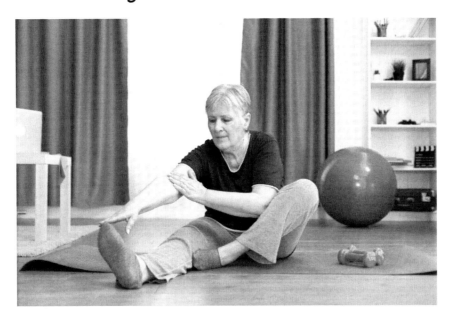

By increasing your flexibility, you'll increase the range of motion in each of your joints and find that moving around is easier. All those daily movements will seem much easier, and you'll feel free of painful niggles. Your posture and balance will improve, and you'll be less likely to sustain an accident. Additionally, we all understand how amazing it feels to stretch our bodies. Stretching can relieve stress and tension, which promotes a positive outlook, a relaxed body, and a nice sensation.

Stretching Eases Arthritis and Low Back Discomfort

Osteoarthritis and spinal stenosis are prominent causes of lower back discomfort in older persons. The most prevalent type of arthritis, osteoarthritis, is brought on by the deterioration of the cartilage in the facet joints over time. Usually, the accompanying low back discomfort is intermittent, but osteoarthritis may lead to sciatica over time. In addition to osteoarthritis of the low back, arthritis commonly manifests in the neck, fingers, toes, hips, and knees. 33.6 percent (12.4 million) of persons 65 and older have osteoarthritis. Spinal stenosis is the narrowing of the bone channel through which the spinal nerves or cord travel. Sciatica signs include tingling, weakness, and numbness in the low back, buttocks, and legs caused by spinal nerve compression.

While osteoarthritis and spinal stenosis are both inevitable aging conditions and cannot be prevented, the pain they cause can be controlled with stretching exercises. Seniors benefit from regular stretching by increasing their range of motion, suppleness, and flexibility to reduce stiffness in the affected joints. Understandably, stretching or moving these joints may be uncomfortable and challenging. Before stretching, it is advised to warm up tense muscles with a heat pack to help with pain management. Conversely, after exercising, it is advised to cool down muscles with an ice pack to help with joint swelling. You could also want to think about assisted stretching with a piece of stretching equipment or another person.

Stretching Reduces the Risk of Falling

For older adults, defined as those 65 and older, the danger of falling is a big worry. One in three senior citizens will fall annually, with 2.5 million people needing emergency room care. According to research, stretching is important for maintaining stability and balance, which helps prevent falls. To reduce falls in older persons, it is crucial to increase hip joint mobility and hamstring, quadriceps, and lower back flexibility.

Stretching Helps Improve Poor Posture

Our body's connective tissue, including ligaments and tendons, loses water as we age, making it less elastic and flexible. Poor posture develops over time due to ligament and tendon tightening in the chest and shoulders and years of slouching at a desk. Forward head position, rounded shoulders, upper back, and forward-pressing hips characterize poor posture. The organic s-curve of our spine compresses. Pain between the shoulder blades and the lower back may result from this.

Consistent stretching is a simple way to increase flexibility. You will have more range of motion, helping to loosen tight ligaments, tendons, and muscles. Additionally, senior strength training routines and a stretching regimen will assist balance out weaker muscles and improve flexibility while correcting poor posture.

Stretching Promotes Energy and Blood Flow

Dynamic stretching is a low intensity stretching method that uses movement to stretch your muscles, versus static stretching, which calls for holding your body stationary while you stretch. Your muscles will lengthen due to dynamic stretches, which also increase the body's blood flow and nutritional absorption. Increasing the body's energy levels. For older people to maintain their independence, remain active in their social networks, and age generally well, they need to feel more vital.

CHAPTER 2: WARM-UP EXERCISES

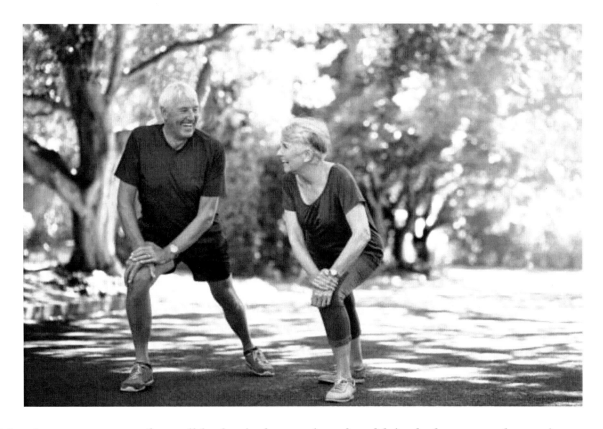

A 10-minute warm-up for mild physical exercise should include some dynamic stretching motions that are appropriate for the activity you're about to conduct and some light aerobic activity.

Contrary to popular belief, there is minimal proof that static stretching lowers the risk of injury during exercise, physical activity, or even pain the following day. Dynamic stretching is still highly well-liked as part of an aerobic warm-up.

Marching

March on the spot at first, then move forward and backward. Keep your elbows bent and your fists relaxed as you raise and lower your arms in time with your feet.

Heel Digs

While keeping the front foot pointed, alternate heels to the front and strike out after each heel dig. Keep the supporting leg slightly bent.

Knee Lifts

Stand tall and raise your alternate knees until they contact the other hand to perform knee lifts. Maintain a firm core and a straight back. Keep the supporting leg slightly bent.

Shoulder Rolls

Continue marching still for shoulder rolls. Roll your shoulders five times forward and five times backward. Arms should be relaxed and at your sides.

Knee Bends

Stand upright to perform knee bends with your feet shoulder-width apart and your hands outstretched. You can lower yourself by no more than 10 cm by bending your knees. As you ascend, repeat.

CHAPTER 3: COOL DOWN EXERCISES

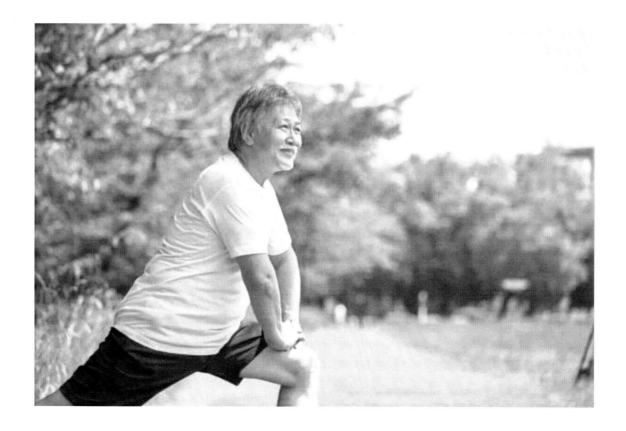

Child's Pose

Kneel on the ground. Next, bend your knees and sit on the back of your calf muscles while keeping your legs together. Put a pillow between the back of your thighs and calves if you cannot drop to your calves to relieve pressure on your knees. After that, fold yourself over the front of your thighs while maintaining touch with your calves and thighs by lowering your head and stretching out with your arms. You'll feel a greater stretch as you extend your reach.

Single Knee-To-Chest Stretch

Bend one knee while lying on your back with your legs straight. Draw the bent knee toward your stomach and chest. Until you experience a stretch in your back, hold your leg with both hands on either the back of your thigh or the shin, whichever position is more comfortable for you. Switch legs after 30 seconds of holding.

Seated Pigeon

On your left knee, place your right ankle while seated on a bench or chair, then slowly push your right knee down. Then, switch to the other leg and hold for another 30 seconds. This will aid in avoiding tightness in your inner thighs.

Standing Quad Stretch

As you raise your left ankle to meet your butt while standing on your right leg, grip your shoe with your left hand. Hold for a minute. The front of your thigh ought to feel stretched. Concentrate on extending your knee as far as possible to maximize the effect. On the right side, repeat.

CHAPTER 4: STRETCHING EXERCISES

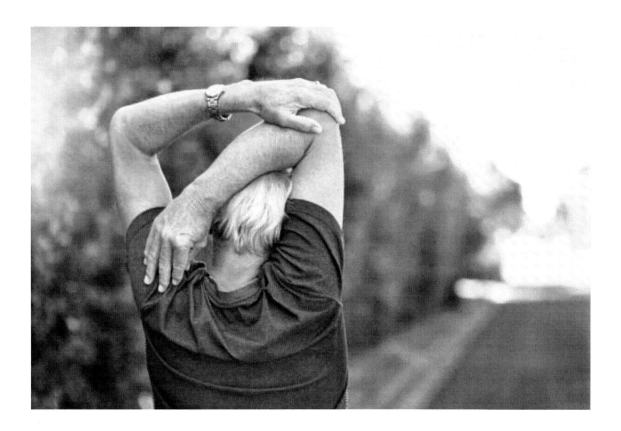

Upper Body Stretches

Neck Stretch

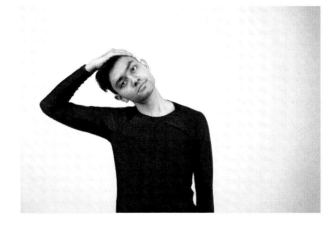

It increases neck mobility and enables you to drive with a wider field of vision. Straighten your back as you stand or sit. If it is comfortable, tilt your head to the left, so your left ear is next to your left shoulder. Pulling your head gently toward your left shoulder requires you to extend your left hand above your head. Up to 30 seconds of holding, then gradually release. Change sides and then repeat.

Shoulder Stretch

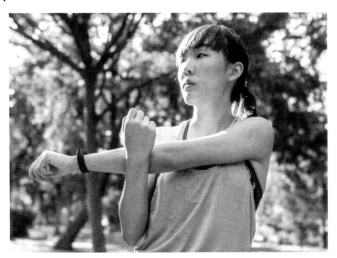

With your chest raised and your back straight. Hold your left arm near your right elbow while bringing your right arm across your body and holding it there. Up to 30 seconds of holding, then gradually release. Seniors should perform shoulder stretches on both sides.

Shoulder Rolls

Better posture while easing shoulder stress and alleviating neck stiffness. Place your arms at your sides when standing or sitting. Inhale, raise your shoulders toward the ceiling and lower them while pulling your shoulder blades closer together. Roll your shoulders back while doing little circles with them. Roll your shoulders opposite for the same reps after repeating them 10-20 times.

Overhead Stretch

It is great for loosening the arm muscles and opening your shoulders. Straighten your spine as you stand or sit, then entwine your fingers with your palms facing downward. Inhale deeply as you extend your arms above your head, turning your palms forward to face the ceiling. Up to 30 seconds, hold. When you are back in your starting posture, exhale. This stretch is good for opening and releasing your shoulders, back, and core.

Upper Back Stretch

Good for stretching minor muscles to enhance the health of the spine and shoulders. Put your hands together in a circle in front of you while standing or sitting. Bring your chin up against your chest. Push through the opposing hand, focusing on opening up your shoulder blades. Senior back stretches hold for up to 30 seconds.

Chest Stretch

It's good for opening the shoulders and chest and helps correct hunched posture. Stretch your arms straight in front of you with your thumbs pointing upward as you stand or sit up straight. Move your arms out and back while maintaining their straightness and parallelism to the ground. Seniors should perform chest stretches after holding for up to 30 seconds.

Side Stretch

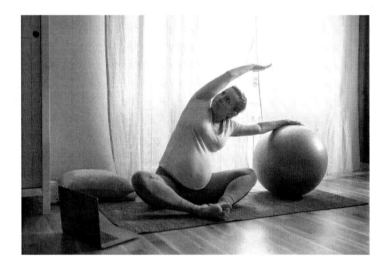

Straighten your spine when standing or sitting, then raise your hands in front of your head. Engage your core muscles as far to the left as you can. Up to 30 seconds, hold. Alternate sides, then repeat.

Overhead Side Stretch

An excellent and simple exercise to relax your stomach, back, and shoulders is the overhead side stretch, also known as the standing side stretch. Standing with your feet shoulder-width apart, extend your arms above your head while, if desired, interlocking your fingers. Leaning slightly to the left while maintaining a long torso. Return to the middle after holding this stretch for 10 to 30 seconds. Repeat the stretch on the right side. You can perform this workout while seated. Similar techniques can be used to perform this exercise for older people with mobility or health issues.

Keep your hips, knees, and toes pointed forward while seated high in a chair. Repeat the instructions above while raising your arms above your head. (If you find this challenging, put your arms down by your sides or on your hips.) For ten to thirty seconds, gently lean to one side.

Trunk Stretch

Good for: strengthening and reducing back discomfort while also increasing blood flow to the lower back for everyday functional activities like bending or twisting. Sit up or stand straight to cross your arms over your chest. Try to solely rotate your trunk while you twitch to the right as far as is comfortable. Up to 30 seconds, hold. It should be repeated after switching sides.

Shoulder Flexion

You can elongate your shoulders with this quick shoulder stretch. Shoulder joint that can be used to treat and stop muscle degeneration. With your opposing hand, grab one of your arms and slowly, delicately drag it across your chest until you feel a stretch in your shoulder. (be sure to maintain your elbow below shoulder height while stretching.) Hold this posture for ten to thirty seconds, then switch to the opposite arm. To get the most out of your stretching exercises, you can perform this stretch while standing or sitting, depending on your preference.

Triceps Stretch

The triceps stretch comes next but is final for our upper body. The triceps stretch, intended to stretch your arms, is a terrific technique to increase your shoulder mobility. The triceps stretch is similar to the rest of our upper body workouts in that it may be done standing or sitting. Just be sure to sit up straight and support your back with a chair!

Put your feet hip-width apart and hold yourself up straight. Raise your right arm behind your head while raising both arms above your head. After that, place your left hand on your right elbow and slowly draw it towards your back until you feel your upper arm expanding. Repeat this stretch with your left arm, holding it for 10 to 30 seconds. Then, bring your arms back to their starting positions.

Lower Body Stretches

Standing Quadriceps Stretch

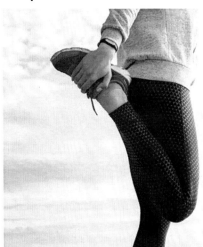

Your knees and hips will be more mobile after performing the knee-to-chest stretch exercise. The standing quadriceps stretch is the first exercise on our list. The standing quadriceps stretch is a fantastic exercise for seniors as it is essential for mobility and flexibility. Since the legs are the largest extremities, several stretches may be necessary to reap their full health advantages. The quadriceps muscle, which is situated on the top portion of your upper leg, is the focus of this exercise.

As you will be balancing on one leg for this exercise, grab the back of a chair or a couch for support. Better support is heavier support. With your left hand, cling to the chair. With your right hand holding your leg by the ankle, gently draw your right foot toward your bottom while bending your right knee. For a period of 10 to 30 seconds, maintain this posture. Then, lower your leg again and repeat with your left leg. You might attempt the seated ankle stretch, which is excellent for stretching your quadriceps if you have trouble standing up. Because it affects more than just your legs, this lower body stretch is an important workout for seniors.

Similar to the previous workout, warm up your legs by taking a short walk to limber them a bit. Sit comfortably in your chair, then, with your right hand, slowly draw your right knee toward your chest. Hold this position for 10 to 30 seconds once you start to feel the stretching. Repeat this exercise with your second leg, gently lowering it to the floor.

Ankle Circles

Take a straight stance with your feet hip-width apart and your arms by your sides. Point your left toe downward and shift your weight to your right leg. Make a little circle with your ankles while rotating your left foot. Use your right foot to perform the exercise once more. To widen your ankle joints as much as possible, start with smaller circles and gradually increase their diameter. Return to smaller circles if you experience any pain or discomfort. Keep your breathing calm and your movements fluid.

Hamstring Stretch

Now that your quadriceps and hips have been addressed, it's time to give your hamstrings a little attention. This stretching exercise concentrates on your legs and lowers your back, which is important for seniors to retain flexibility. This stretch will maintain your legs and back flexible and loose while reducing stiffness.

Choose a stable surface to sit on. Next, extend a leg outward onto the ground. Reach for your thigh, knee, or ankle as you slowly lean forward and inhale. (Take care not to overextend your hamstring during this stretch.) Next, maintain this position for 10 to 30 seconds, gently place your leg back on the floor, and then switch to the opposite side of your body to repeat.

Soleus Stretch

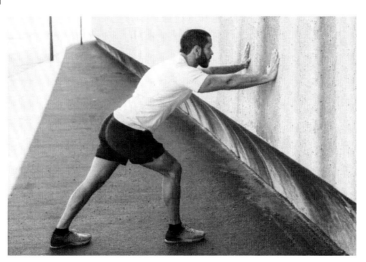

The calf muscle, another important leg muscle group, benefits greatly from this straightforward stretch. The soleus stretch targets your calves and lower body flexibility by enhancing the deep calf muscle and the general usability of your legs.

To begin this stretching activity: as you confront a wall, stand up. Put your right foot in front of your left and support yourself by resting both hands on the wall. Once you're at ease, start softly bending your knees until your lower leg feels stretched. For ten to thirty seconds, maintain this posture. Slowly rise once you've had a chance to stretch and feel good. Then, switch the locations of your left and right feet and perform the exercise again.

Chair Lunge

Try this stretching exercise for seniors to preserve your mobility and muscle strength. However, because it can be challenging, this practice is not required. Make sure to only do this work out if your body tells you to.

While standing with the chair behind you, put your right shin on the chair's seat. The next step is slightly bending your front left leg while pulling your hips down and forward. Hold this position for 10 to 30 seconds, then switch to the other side and repeat.

Advanced Standing Hip Flexor

This stretch, one of many hip flexor exercises for seniors, is excellent for releasing tightness or soreness in your hips. It should be noted that this is a challenging exercise and might be more appropriate for people with greater experience. Grab a sturdy chair, then stand with your feet facing the back of it. Make sure you are far enough away from the chair so that you can pull your leg up. Then, while still holding on to the chair with both hands, lift the opposite leg toward your chest while bending the knee and bringing it as close to your chest as you can. Hold this posture for ten to fifteen seconds, then switch to the other leg.

Hamstring Stretch

With your feet shoulder-width apart, stand erect. Bend your left leg and extend your right foot in front of you. Put your hands on your right upper thigh while slowly hinging at the hips, then slowly depress. Up to 30 seconds, hold. Repeat the hamstring stretch after switching sides.

With Chair

Place your right leg in front of you with the heel still on the floor as you lean toward the edge of your chair. Slowly extend your arm, bending at the hips but maintaining a straight back. Up to 30 seconds, hold. Seniors should alternate sides and then perform hamstring stretches.

Piriformis Stretch

It reduces knee and ankle discomfort. Helps with sciatic discomfort as well. Cross your left leg slowly over your right leg as you lean forward in your chair. Maintaining a straight back, lean forward as far as is comfortable. Up to 30 seconds, hold. Stretches for seniors on a chair: alternate sides, then repeat.

Calf Stretch

Place both hands against the wall in front of you while keeping your arms fully extended as you face the wall and step back a few inches. Leaning against the wall, extend your right leg behind you while bending your left leg. Bring your hips forward as you drive your right heel into the ground. Up to 30 seconds, hold. The stretch should be repeated after switching sides.

Seated

Reducing ankle joint stiffness, which might prevent potential falls. Wrap a towel around the toes of your left foot as you sit down. Your left leg should be extended forward with your heel on the ground. Hold and gently pull the towel for up to 20 seconds. Change sides and then repeat.

Chair Stretches For Back Pain

According to the American Chiropractic Association, back discomfort is the second most common cause of doctor visits (ACA). Back discomfort can result from arthritic conditions, excess weight carried about, bad posture, and even physiological stress. In reality, according to the ACA, most cases of back pain are mechanical, meaning an infection, a fracture, or any other grave conditions do not bring them on. Back discomfort caused by internal issues like kidney stones or blood clots is less frequent.

This indicates that treating or preventing back pain at home may be a good alternative. More than that, maintaining strong postural muscles, a flexible spine, and continuing to move in supported ways are some of the best strategies to completely avoid back discomfort, especially as we age. Simple stretching can accomplish all of this. Before performing these stretches, or if you are already experiencing back pain, consult your doctor or physical therapist.

All the exercises listed here should be performed while seated in a strong chair, preferably not an armchair but a large dining room chair. If you're sitting on a firmer surface, it will be simpler to maintain good posture. No other tools are needed. Make sure you sit squarely in the seat, not perched on the edge, with your feet firmly planted and your knees bent at a 90-degree angle.

Neck and Chest Stretch

Before screens became so common in our lives, people usually jutted their chins forward or downward to read, eat, drive, and do other activities. In addition to causing neck discomfort, this can aggravate pain in the upper and middle back and other spine areas. The following exercise helps relieve this discomfort while stretching out the chest, which can feel constrained due to poor posture and needs to be opened back up.

This softly exercises your obliques while stretching your pectorals, erector spinae, scapulae, and trapezius muscles in your neck. Starting seated, place your feet flat on the floor and sit up straight. With your fingers entwined and your thumbs extending by your ears and down your neck, place your hands at the base of your skull. (With your head resting in your hands, this is the traditional "relaxed, laid back" stance.) Turn your face forward while easing your head back into your hands.

Deeply inhale. When you exhale, relax your left elbow so that it is pointing further downward and your right elbow so that it is pointing upward. Your neck will stretch in a supportive manner as a result. Observation: Since this should be a simple motion, it's okay if your elbows barely travel a few inches. It shouldn't hurt, just feel like a good stretch. Take two long breaths, then slowly bring your spine back to neutral. Repeat on the opposite side, the right elbow pointing down and the left elbow pointing up. Each side should be repeated three times, swapping sides each time.

Seated Gentle Backbend

Because of our chins sticking out or falling, as previously indicated, as well as how we usually make this motion throughout our lives, as we get older, our upper and midback (the thoracic and cervical spine) start to bend forward even more. Instead of being our "lazy" posture, it can become our normal posture. This can induce strain in our back muscles and contribute to the hunch we usually associate with aging. This easy backbend might help release that tension. During this stretch, your pectorals, anterior neck muscles, and spinal extensors are all worked.

Starting from a seated position with your feet flat on the floor, bring your hands to your lower back, thumbs wrapping around your hips in the direction of your front torso. Inhale while firmly pressing your hands into your lower back and hips. Gently arch your spine, exhale, and tilt your head up, so your face faces the ceiling. The upper and middle spine should bend during the backbend. Take five full deep breaths. Return slowly and gently to the starting position, then repeat three to five times.

Reach Back

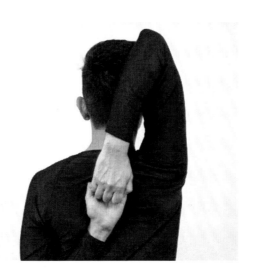

This exercise stretches your chest and shoulders while improving your shoulder range of motion. It can feel comfortable to lean forward while standing or hunch over while sitting. However, pulling those muscles in causes stress in our chests. It might also hurt our upper and midbacks if those muscles aren't used. The technique below enhances shoulder stretch, opens the chest, and trains the postural muscles. Your pectorals, as well as your anterior deltoids, receive a beautiful stretch.

Sit upright with your feet firmly on the ground. Reach your back with your hands and try to interlace them while you take a deep breath. Take a deep breath and feel your spine lengthen as you sit up straighter. Move your shoulder blades down your back while rolling your shoulders up and back.

If your hands are clasped, release them as you exhale and softly straighten your arms. Your upper back will open up as a result.

- Release your clasp and switch back to neutral after taking three long breaths.
- Do this three times.
- Take it a step farther

If everything seems comfortable and there are no signs of tension, you can extend the stretch to include the entire spine. It can help decrease back pain in other areas and improve spinal mobility.

Start by performing the stretch mentioned above while assuming the position with your hands behind your back or grabbing the opposing wrists or elbows.

You'll feel your ribs rising and your spine lengthening as you inhale. Lean forward at the waist as if bringing your ribs to your thighs while maintaining the sensation in your spine.

Continue doing it only as far as it feels comfortable. Do not fall onto your legs, even if you can reach your thighs. To maintain this position and stretch your chest, shoulders, and back, you should continue to use your postural muscles.

Seated Cat-Cow

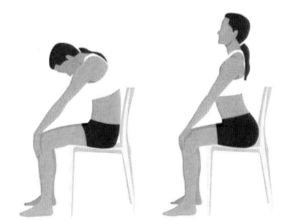

Frequently, discomfort is felt in the lower back. Osteoarthritis and spinal degeneration become significantly more prevalent as we age. Some of us usually stand with a "flat pelvis" when our posture is bad, which can result in significant lower back pain. By strengthening parts of the core muscles and stretching the lower back muscles, the Cat-Cow exercise helps maintain the spine's health.

Your serratus anterior, erector spinae, iliac rib muscle, external abdominal oblique, and rectus abdominis all work and stretch in this combo of two poses.

Keep your feet on the ground firmly and your knees at a 90-degree angle. Place your hands on your knees with your fingers pointing inward and your heel on the outside of the legs.

Exhale while pressing your hands into the floor and arching your back completely. As a result, you should feel like you're pressing your butt out from behind you while facing the sky.

Roll your shoulders forward as you breathe in again, bring your belly button in toward your spine, tuck your chin into your chest, and push with your hands toward your knees.

Reverse the motion on your subsequent exhalation by pulling your chest through your arms, arching your spine once more, and pressing down into your legs rather than your knees.

Three to five times, gently and while breathing in and out.

Gentle Twist

Gently twisting your spine is one of the greatest stretches for lower back pain and offers several advantages, such as improving digestion and circulation and toning your abs. Additionally, performing a gentle twist a few times per day might assist in maintaining spinal flexibility and prevent future lower back pain.

This stretch engages your serratus anterior, erector spinae, rhomboids, and other neck muscles (such as sternocleidomastoid and splenius capitis). Once more, begin with your feet firmly on the ground, and your knees bent at a 90-degree angle. On the seat, lean slightly forward. You need a little extra space behind you but don't want to feel unsteady or like the chair might tilt forward.

Put pressure on your seat, sit straight, stretch your spine, and raise your arms as you breathe. Exhale and turn slightly to the right, placing your right hand wherever it feels comfortable and your left hand on the outside of your right knee. Avoid using that hand to "crank" your twist deeper by placing it anywhere other than the seat or back of the chair. Using your arm strength to twist yourself more forcefully can hurt you and cause one part of your spine to twist more forcefully than the other; you want to feel the twist equally throughout your entire spine.

Continue to twist, and as you breathe in, notice how much taller you are sitting. Twist a little bit more as you exhale.

Before gently releasing the twist and repeating it on the opposite side, take three to five deep breaths. Stretch at least twice on each side as you alternate.

Seated Rotation

The torso's muscles, including the back and abs, are worked during seated rotations. Hold a medicine ball or weight (for example a bottle of water) while sitting in your chair. Hold the weight with your elbows out to the sides, shoulders relaxed, and it should be at chest level. Rotate the torso to the right while keeping the knees and hips pointing forward. Pay attention to contracting the muscles in your waist area. Keep the rotation slow and controlled as you turn to the left, then back to the center. For 12 reps, continue switching sides. Twists to the right and left are combined into one rep.

CHAPTER 5: ROUTINE EXERCISES

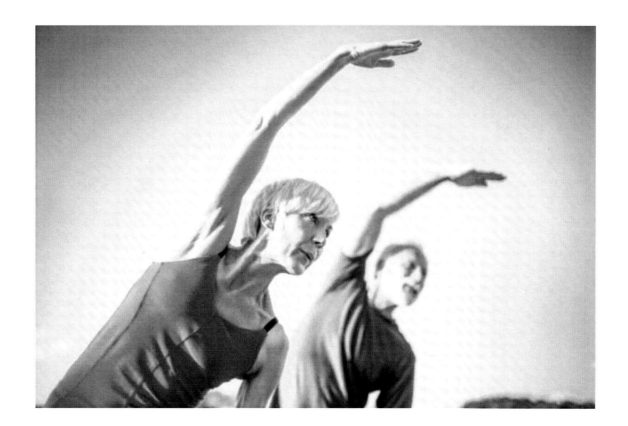

Everyday Morning Routine

Wake up every morning and follow this routine to relax different body parts. This morning routine can be carried out within just 15 minutes. Besides the suggested warm-ups, you can also try walking for 5-10 minutes to activate your muscles.

Warm-Up

1. **Marching:** 3 minutes
2. **Heel Digs:** 60 seconds
3. **Knee lifts:** 60 seconds

Workout

1. **Neck Stretch:** 10 reps
2. **Shoulder Stretch:** 10 reps
3. **Side Stretch:** 8 reps on each side
4. **Ankle Circles:** 10 reps
5. **Seated Gentle backbend:** 10 reps
6. **Seated Cat-Cow:** 12 reps

Cool Down

1. **Seated Pigeon:** 60 seconds
2. **Single knee to chest stretch:** 60 seconds

Note: While doing the stretches, ensure you are not overstraining your muscles. Be slow and gentle. If you have any medical condition affecting bones and muscles, consult your physiotherapist before trying these stretches.

Back Pain Tension Routine

This 15-minute routine can help relieve back pain; it is useful to decompress your spine and give it an upright posture. Breathe in and out while repeating each stretch in the routine.

Warm-Up

1. **Knee lifts:** 3 minutes
2. **Marching:** 60 seconds
3. **Knee bends:** 10 reps

Workout

1. **Shoulder Rolls:** 10 reps
2. **Upper Back Stretch:** 10 reps
3. **Chest Stretch:** 20 reps
4. **Seated Gentle backbend:** 20 reps
5. **Gentle Twist:** 10 reps
6. **Seated Cat Cow:** 20 reps
7. **Seated Rotation:** 20 reps

Cool Down

1. **Child's Pose:** 60 seconds
2. **Seated Pigeon:** 60 seconds

Note: Do not go overboard with the seated rotation; rotate slowly to repeat the move.

Neck Pain Resolution Routine

Neck pain is common among adults and can be treated with regular stretches. Combining the neck stretch with the following warm-up routine can ease neck strain.

Warm-Up

1. **Shoulder rolls:** 2 sets of 10 reps
2. **Marching:** 3 minutes

Workout

1. **Neck Stretch:** 12 reps on each side
2. **Reach Back:** 10 reps
3. **Overhead stretch:** 12 reps

Cool Down

1. **Single Knee-To-Chest Stretch:** 60 seconds
2. **Child's Pose:** 60 seconds

Note: Rub the back of your neck gently for 1 minute after the exercise or use warm compresses to soothe the muscles and increase the blood flow.

Legs Exercises Routine

This leg stretches routine relieves your quadriceps and hamstrings after a hectic day. It is particularly useful for desk or table work all day.

Warm-Up

1. **Marching**: 3 minutes
2. **Heel Digs**: 60 seconds
3. **Knee lifts**: 30 seconds

Workout

1. **Standing quadriceps stretch:** 10 reps
2. **Hamstring stretch:** 10 reps
3. **Soleus Stretch:** 10 reps
4. **Chair Lunge:** 10 reps
5. **Calf Stretch:** 10 reps

Cool Down

1. **Child's Pose:** 60 seconds
2. **Standing Quad Stretch:** 60 seconds

Note: Warm compresses work well to relax the pulled muscles. Keep the reps to 10 for each exercise if you are a beginner.

Posture Enhancement Routine

If you want to prevent slouching or get rid of it, this routine can slowly help you improve your posture. You can carry out this routine any time of the day as long as you have 10-15 minutes to spare for it.

Warm-Up

1. **Marching:** 3 minutes
2. **Shoulder rolls:** 60 seconds
3. **Knee lifts:** 30 seconds

Workout

1. **Trunk Stretch:** 10 reps
2. **Side Stretch:** 10 reps
3. **Shoulder Flexion:** 10 reps
4. **Standing Quadriceps Stretch:** 10 reps
5. **Upper Back Stretch:** 10 reps
6. **Seated Cow-Cat:** 10 reps

Cool Down

1. **Child's Pose:** 60 seconds
2. **Single Knee-To-Chest Stretch:** 60 seconds

Note: Take a 30 second break between each exercise. Avoid overstraining your muscles by stretching too much.

Advanced Stretch Workout

If you want to work on your entire body's muscles, then this advanced workout can help. As you progress, you can increase the reps for each stretch but make sure to divide the total workout duration evenly between all the stretches

Warm-Up
1. **Marching:** 10 minutes

Workout
1. **Reach Back:** 20 Reps
2. **Seated Gentle Backbend:** 20 reps
3. **Piriformis stretch:** 15 reps
4. **Hamstring stretch:** 15 reps
5. **Side Stretch:** 10 reps
6. **Shoulder Flexion:** 15 reps

Cool Down
1. **Seated Pigeon:** 60 seconds
2. **Single Knee-To-Chest Stretch:** 60 seconds

Note: Take a 30 second break between each stretch. Inhale deeply and try to relax while stretching.

BOOK 3:
CORE AND BALANCE EXERCISE FOR SENIORS

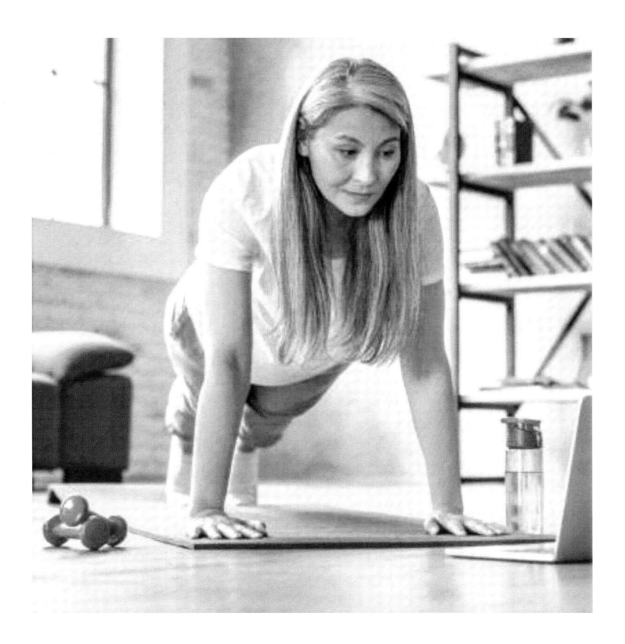

CHAPTER 1: CORE AND BALANCE EXERCISES

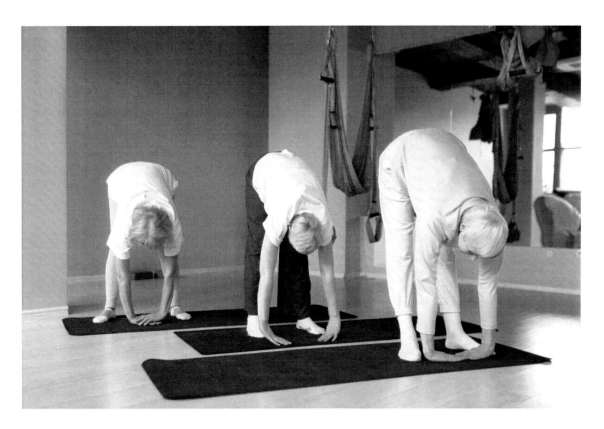

Our core muscles support our spine, improve agility, and facilitate daily movement. As a result, we are less prone to encounter falls caused by poor balance. Many people mistakenly believe that the abdominal muscles are part of the core. The entire torso is comprised of the core muscles, which do include the abdominals. The main parts are made up of the following:

- The abdominis rectus (the front stomach muscles)
- The obliques, both internal and exterior (the muscles running along the sides)
- Transverse abdominal muscle (the layer of muscle surrounding the spine)
- Those in the hips
- Those in the lower back

Age-Related Core Strength

As early as our mid-30s, our core muscular tissue naturally starts to atrophy! So, it becomes increasingly necessary as we age to improve on our core strengths. Core muscle fibers weaken and lose some of their flexibility over time if you don't perform regular core strength exercises. Additionally, since our core muscles mostly support our spine, weakness in these muscles makes us more vulnerable to injuries. A weak core generally increases the chance of falling and becoming hurt due to poor balance and restricted movement.

Seniors Need to Build Core Strength

Everyone should have a strong core, but seniors, in particular, should pay special attention because a weak core can contribute significantly to injuries. Avoiding injuries is essential for this age group since, as we age, the recovery process becomes more time-consuming and challenging. The Centers for Disease Control and Prevention estimate that millions of Americans 65 years of age and older fall annually. More concerning is that one in five falls results in serious injuries. Maintaining core strength is essential for elders to prevent falls.

- Strengthening: research has shown that seniors' bodies can become stronger with core strengthening exercises.

- Balance is improved by using your core to support your spine, which helps with stability and posture.

- Making routine jobs simpler: everyday activities like getting out of bed, getting out of a chair, and mounting stairs include the core muscles. These regular tasks are easier when you have a strong core.

- Avoiding, controlling, and minimizing back pain: your likelihood of developing back discomfort increases as you age, particularly in the lower back. A strong core will help avoid back discomfort because the lower back is a part of the core. Core exercises will stretch and strengthen these muscles for seniors with lower back discomfort, which will assist in lessening the pain. Maintaining a strong core can help people with no back problems avoid developing it.

- Seniors can benefit from these advantages by including core strengthening activities in their fitness regimen.

Core Stability and Life Quality

The way you move every day, in every situation, is influenced by your core muscles. The core connects our upper body and lower body as the center of our body. Our ability to lift, reach, pivot, and bend is impacted. Any movement, no matter how modest, can be sustained by our spine thanks to the stability of our core muscles. Core stability is needed for everything from cleaning the house and playing with the grandchildren to taking a walk and operating a vehicle. Without it, there is a higher chance of injury when performing daily duties.

When we carry out everyday tasks like standing up straight and walking with good balance, we may not be aware of our core muscles' role. However, these activities may become challenging if these muscles start to deteriorate. The significance of the core to our general well-being and quality of life is then cruelly made clear. For better or worse, core strength and stability significantly affect senior citizens' quality of life. In the end, a solid core supports a sound back, which guards against discomfort and damage. Additionally, it increases stability and balance to lower your chance of falling.

Therefore, you should prioritize maintaining a strong core if you want to stay healthy, continue your regular activities with ease, and help prevent accidents from falls. Remember to consult your doctor to be sure you can perform them safely before including them in your regular fitness program.

Signs of a Weak Core

You already know how crucial it is to have a strong core because it is the basis for your body's motions. A strong midsection will help you get the most out of your workouts and make it simpler for you to carry out daily duties and prevent injuries.

Your Posture isn't On Point

Your core might not function properly if you see yourself slouching at a poor desk or noticing your posture when you glance at yourself in the mirror. Your posture can become crooked if your core muscles are weak.

You Can't Do the "Stand Up" Test

Sitting on the floor is one of the simplest ways to assess your core strength. You probably need to do more core exercises if you can't stand up without resting your hands on the floor or your knees. This test accurately predicts core strength, mobility, stability, and coordination for all ages.

Your Lower Back Hurts

If a back injury has been ruled out as the source of your lower back pain, your weak core may be to blame for your post-workout stiffness and soreness. When your core isn't stable enough, even the smallest change might put unnecessary pressure on your spine and increase your risk of injury.

You Have Balance Issues

Your core may be partially to blame if you struggle with the standing series in your

monthly yoga practice. When you move, especially when you make quick motions like turning or twisting, your core muscles balance your body.

Benefits of Core Training

It Supports Better Posture

Having stronger core muscles, especially the inner core muscles that attach to your spine, will help you maintain excellent posture and stand up straighter.

It Enhances Equilibrium

Your balance benefits from having a strong overall core and the good posture it promotes. That's because it's simpler to maintain your balance on uneven ground or get back up after falling when you start from a strong base. Your body achieves homeostasis as a result. You have a little more height and equilibrium throughout your entire body.

It Encourages Proper Walking Form

Another benefit of improved balance? A strong core also helps you maintain good form as you walk. With less rocking and wasted energy, the pelvis, hips, and lower back can function more harmoniously when the core is strong. That bodes well for your upcoming walk, but consistent use of the proper technique can also help you log those miles without strain or injury.

It Makes Things More Stable

A strong torso aids in balance maintenance during every exercise. You can stand up straighter and keep your trunk steady when exercising or doing your daily activities if you have a strong core. Your risk of muscular strains, lower back pain, and slouching are all significantly increased by a weak core.

It Safeguards Your Organs

Your body's organs play a crucial role in its operation, and a solid core can assist some of them in staying secure. Your abdominal wall, a barrier between you and the outside world, is home to many organs, including your liver, spleen, kidneys, and more. As a result, the better your core is built, the better it will shield that tissue from force or harm from the outside world.

It Simplifies Day-to-Day Life

All your movements start at your core. Therefore, the simpler it is to carry out daily actions like bending over to pick up something off the ground, standing for extended periods, or performing household tasks, the stronger your core is. Due to their ability to make you more functional, many core exercises fall under functional fitness. They can make it easier for you to go about your day.

It Can Lessen or Stop the Pain

Another significant benefit of a solid core? You feel better all-around as a result. Simply said, having a solid core improves your quality of life. It eases any discomfort you might be experiencing, supports your lower back, strengthens your spine, and generally improves your mood. This is because having a strong core has knock-on consequences that can help you prevent annoyance and lessen the discomfort. These effects include better posture, greater balance, and the ability to move around more easily.

It Encourages Resistance Training

Working the muscles throughout your body can help you perform at your best. Strength is not just vital in your core. Additionally, having a strong core prepares you for success with added strength training. The capacity to lift more weight increases with core strength.

Do you want to add some core exercises to your daily regimen? These core exercises are simple and they were created for your activity level with seniors in mind.

CHAPTER 2: WARM-UP AND COOL-DOWN EXERCISES

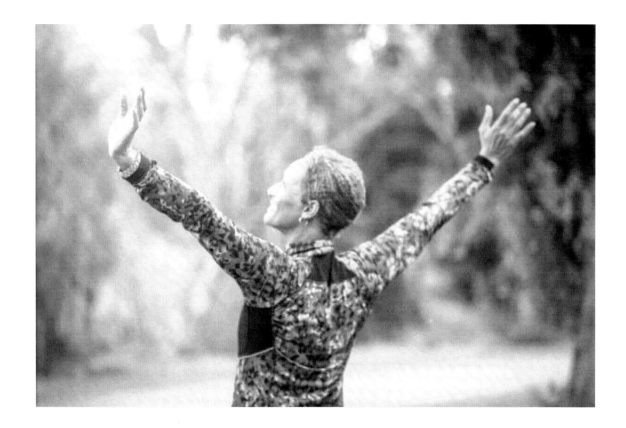

Warm Up

Just before you intend to begin your workout, warm up. Start your warm-up by concentrating on your hamstrings and other big muscle groups. Start by engaging in the movement patterns and activities associated with your preferred exercise, but at a slow pace that progressively picks up speed and intensity. It's known as a dynamic warmup. Warming up may cause light perspiration, but it won't usually make you feel worn out.

- Take a moderate stroll for five to ten minutes to warm up.

Standing Criss-Cross Crunches

Put your hands behind your head and stand with your feet hip-width apart. Lift your right knee as high as possible while bending your right leg. Bring your right knee near your left elbow while turning your torso to the right. When the set is finished, repeat on the opposing side and alternate sides continuously.

Standing Side Crunch

Bring your left knee near your left elbow, shift your weight to your right leg, and crunch to the left side. Repeat while changing legs.

Alternating Toe Touches

Legs should be somewhat broader than shoulder width apart while starting to stand. Touch with your left hand your right toes while bending your right knee slightly, then return to your starting posture while raising your arms to your sides in a T shape. Repeat touching your right hand to your left toes.

Alternating Side Lunge

Step with your left leg to the side while keeping your right leg straight. Touch your left foot with your right hand. Repeat the motion on the right side.

Back Rolls

Begin by sitting upright, knees bent, and feet pointed toward the ceiling. Bring your hands to the front or rear of your shins while keeping your feet firmly on the ground. Rock back onto your shoulders while contracting your abs, then move to your starting posture.

Cooling Down

Standing Forward Bend

While standing, keep your knees straight and attempt to touch the back of your ankles.

Cat/Cow

On the mat or a flat surface start by spreading your fingers widely while on all fours with your hands, feet and knees touching the mat. First inhale and gently arch your back to the ceiling and then exhale lower your stomach towards the ground.

Marching In Place

On the mat or a flat surface, lie down supine. Hold your hands at your sides or above your belly. Take your right leg off the ground while maintaining knee flexion until your thigh and lower leg is at a 90-degree angle. Bring your right knee up to your pelvis. Put your foot down again on the floor. Similarly, move your left foot.

CHAPTER 3: CORE STRENGTH EXERCISES

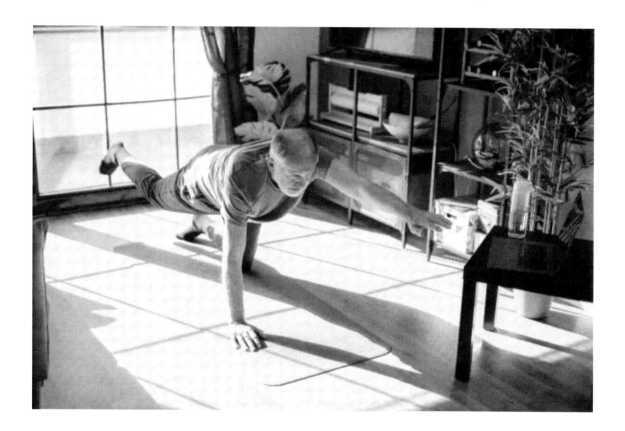

Beginner's Training

Seated Knee-To-Chest

Easily balance yourself at the chair's edge while sitting there. Keep a straight back and a tight core (abdominals, lumbar). Grasp the seat with both hands and place them at the sides of the chair to maintain stability. Both feet should be placed in front of the torso with the toes facing up. Gently bring both legs up toward the torso, bending the knees. With both knees, get as close to the chest as you can. Slowly return to the beginning position by performing this action in the exact opposite direction. One "rep" is equal to this. One leg at a time is another way to isolate this movement. Before lifting, just ensure the other side's leg is securely placed on the ground.

Extended Leg Raises

Lay on your back with your legs straight and parallel and your hands touching the floor. Lift your legs as high as possible while keeping them straight. Lower your legs so they are just above the floor. Hold on for a second and return to the starting position. Repeat.

Seated Forward Bends

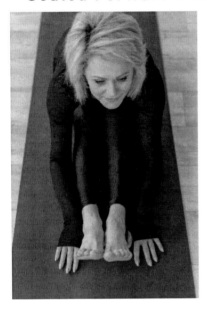

Sit on a mat or a flat surface. Put your hands on your knees with your spine straight and shoulders rolled back. Look directly forward. This is where you start. Bend forward and try to touch your ankles with your hands. After five seconds, release the position and stand back up. Repeat 5 times.

Lying Ankle Tap

Recline on a mat. Keep your knees bent and both of your feet flat on the ground. Keep your hands by your sides and lift your neck slightly off the floor. Now touch the right ankle with your right hand. Go back to the beginning. You bend to the left and try to touch the left ankle with your left hand. Repeat 12 times in total.

Tummy Twists

This core workout can also help to lengthen the spine. For complete abdominal tension, practice this exercise while holding a medicine ball or a comparable object in your hands. Pick up a medicine ball (or similar object). For more space, savor the chair's edge and sit pleasantly there. Keep your lumbar region and abdominals tight. Extend your chest out. With elbows bent, both hands should hold the medicine ball's sides in front of the body. Holding the ball in front of you, lift it a few inches off the lap, and then rotate your upper body to the right. After rotating to the left, return to the center of the body to complete the motion. One complete rotation counts as one "rep."

Side Bends Obliques

With your arms by your sides and feet about shoulder-width apart, start leaning to the right, bringing your right hand's fingers up to your knee. Make sure to maintain your front-facing posture and avoid twisting. Do the same on your left side after you've returned to your starting position. The exercise can also be done while seated in a chair. Reach your right hand down toward your right calf while sitting. Repeat on your left side.

Wood Chops

Stand with your hands clasped tightly in front of you and your feet hip distance apart. Then, in the opposite direction, "chop" your arms up toward your right ear while maintaining a straight arm position. On the other side, repeat. Changes: while seated, lower your arms near your outer right knee. Repeat on your left side after raising your arms back up.

Dead Bug

Knees bowed, lie down supine on the ground. Raise your right leg so your shin is parallel to the floor while maintaining a bent knee. Do the same with your left leg as you bring your right foot back down to the floor. If reclining on the floor is too challenging, you might try a seated knee lift. If you find this too simple, try elevating both legs at once.

Plank

The plank is a fantastic core exercise but a little more difficult than the others on the list. Thus, it is a fantastic objective to strive for. Lay on your stomach and press your forearms firmly into the ground to perform a plank. Squeeze your glutes, quads, and abdominal muscles to lift yourself off the ground while maintaining a straight back. Keep pressing onto your forearms to prevent your lower back and shoulder blades from drooping downward. Try maintaining the position for 10–20 seconds before dropping back to the floor.

You can perform a modified plank from your knees if a plank proves to be too difficult. To avoid sagging and lower back pain, tighten your abdominal muscles. Alternatively, you can perform a standing plank while pressing your hands against a wall.

March with Extended Legs

Lie down supine on the mat or a flat surface. Either place your hands on top of your belly or by your sides. Lift your right leg off the ground to get your lower leg and thigh to meet at a 90-degree angle. Put your foot down again on the floor. Similarly, move your left foot. Ten to fifteen times.

Core Squats for Strength

Place the feet flat on the ground as you lie on the mat with your knees extended. Lift your right leg off the ground while leaving your knee flexed. Bring your right knee up to your pelvis. Your palms should be on the right thigh. Your palms should be pressed up against your thigh. Hold for three seconds, then let go. Place your foot firmly on the ground. The left foot is in the same manner. Ten times total.

Intermediate-Advanced Exercises

Leg Kicks

Easily balance yourself at the chair's edge while sitting there. Maintain a straight back and a tight core (abdominals, lumbar). Grasp the seat with both hands and place them at the sides of the chair to maintain stability. Put both feet in front of you with the toes pointed forward. To the hips, both feet should be diagonal. To stabilize moving both feet forward, softly incline your upper body backward.

Without shifting the body's center, raise one leg as high as possible, aiming to end parallel to the hips. Return the leg to its starting position gradually before switching to the other. Imagine that the person is swimming and kicking their legs in the water as you think about this activity. One "rep" equals one kick per leg. Try not to contact the ground with the feet until the exercise is complete to make it more difficult.

Modified Planks

One of the most well-liked core workouts for people of all ages is the plank. The exercise tightens the core more, causing the body to maintain stability. The ability to maintain proper posture when seated is one benefit of training with this action.

Grasp the sides of the chair with both hands. Move both feet back a few steps so that the body is in front of the chair at a diagonal while maintaining a modest bend in both arms at the elbows. Check whether the back is arched, or the buttocks are raised high. From shoulder to heel, the body should be in a straight line. Seniors are in the right position if they feel resistance (tension) in their core. Keep your body in this position for 30 seconds (or as long as you can without experiencing pain), and then get up or sit down to take a little break. Repeat three or more times. For further stability, lean the chair up against a wall.

Leg Kicks using Resistance Bands

Make a loop at one end of a resistance band by grabbing it. Get on all fours while holding the other end with your right hand and circling your right leg with the loop. Keep your abs and glutes tight and your elbows directly underneath your shoulders. Your right leg should be raised off the ground and extended back so your toes are flat. Take your right foot off the ground. Lift it while keeping it stretched until your spine and leg are parallel. Your foot is downward. Lift it once again just before it touches the ground. Before switching legs, repeat this motion ten times.

Oblique Twists When Seated

Occupy a chair. Maintain a straight back, rolled-back shoulders, and hands resting on your thighs. Take a forward-looking posture. With the elbows out, clasp your hands together in front of your chest. This is where everything begins. Turn your upper body to the right, then to the left, while keeping your eyes forward. Ten to fifteen times.

Seated Side Bends

Occupy a chair. Keep your hands open to the side, your spine upright, and your eyes forward while keeping your feet shoulder-width apart. This is where everything begins. Try to touch the floor with the right hand while bending to the right. Return to standing and slant your left side. Repeat this twelve times.

The Plank Save

Go down on all fours. Put your elbows on the ground while flexing them. Place the toes of your right leg behind you and extend it. Step back with your left leg. On your elbows and toes, support your body. Keep your glutes and core active. Keep holding this position for 10 to 30 seconds while breathing normally. After 30 seconds of relaxation, do it twice more.

Knee Planks

Lay down on your stomach with your elbows bent and your weight on your forearms. Lift the body so that the weight is on the knees and elbows. Maintain the straightest back you can while pushing your stomach into your spine. Avoid letting your hips sag or lift. Remember breathing. Work your way up to 1-2 minutes of holding for 30 seconds. Continue for 1-3 sets.

Knuckle Side Planks

Start by lying on your side with your arms bent and your weight on your elbow. Knees should also be bent. Raise the body so that the elbow and knee bear weight. Maintain as much uprightness as you can. Work your way up to 1-2 minutes of holding for 30 seconds. Repeat for 1-3 sets on each side.

Birddog

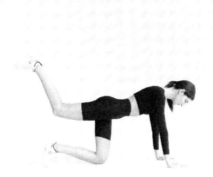

Begin by getting down on all fours with your hands beneath your shoulders and your knees touching the mat. Maintain a straight back and a spine-aligned head. Put out right arm for five seconds. Returning to the starting position, put the right leg out, and hold it there for five seconds. Check that the arm and leg are parallel to the back. If you cannot extend the leg in parallel, you can create a 90-degree angle between your ankle and gluteus. For 1-3 sets, carry out ten repetitions of each leg-and-arm combination.

Crunches

Lay on your back, knees bent, and hands clasped behind your head to start. Elbows ought to be spread wide. Take a deep breath first and, as you exhale, lift your shoulders 6-12 inches off the floor. Look up and avoid tucking your chin down to avoid straining your neck. Hold for a couple of seconds, then restart.

Twisted Crunches

Start in the same spot as a crunch. Turn to the right instead of straight up, then come back to the beginning point.

Twist to the left and then back to the starting position on the following repeat. Perform 1-3 sets of 5-10 repetitions.

Leg Raises

Lay flat on your back with your legs flat to start. For comfort and lower back support, slide your hands under your back. Lift legs slowly, about 12 inches off the ground, and then slowly return to the starting position. If this is challenging, lift one leg at a time until you are strong enough to lift both or flex the knees slightly. Perform 1-3 sets of 10-15 repetitions.

Reverse Crunch

Lay on your back and for one repetition slowly bring both knees close to your chest. For stability, place your hands at your sides flat on the ground. Perform 1-3 sets of 10-15 repetitions.

Traditional Wood Chop

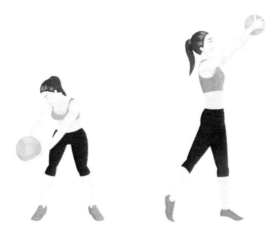

Start with standing with a medicine ball in your hand (4-6 lbs.). Shoulders and legs should be slightly apart. Start by raising the ball above your head. When lowering the ball, flex your knees and move your hips back. As the ball descends to knee height, the arms should remain straight. Keep your knees behind your toes, not in front of them. For 1-3 sets, go back to the beginning position and perform ten repetitions of each. Breathing is important when completing core workouts. Breathe during the release/rest phase and out during the contraction/initial phase.

Advanced Birddog

Begin by getting down on all fours with your hands and knees beneath your shoulders. The right arm and left leg should be raised while maintaining a straight spine and without arching the back. Verify that the arm and leg are parallel to the back. Before returning to the starting position, maintain balance for 5 seconds. For 1-3 sets, carry out ten repetitions of each arm-and-leg combination.

Exercises with Medicine Ball

Twist with a Medicine Ball

Begin with your back raised off the ground (or your feet, for a more advanced action). Twist right and left, bringing the medicine ball to the floor on each side as you do so. Either a quick or slow pace can be used for this practice. Do 1-3 sets of 10-20 repetitions.

Transferring a Core Ball

Hold a ball above your head as you begin. Lift your arms and legs to transfer the ball from your head to your knees or feet.

Transfer from the knees/feet to your chest, then return to the beginning position. Perform 1-3 sets of 8-10 repetitions.

Knee Tucks with Core Ball

Start on all fours with the ball underneath the torso. Move your hands forward slowly

until your feet are off the ground, your thighs are on the ball, your shoulders are upright, and your hands are in a plank position. As the ball glides closer to the arms, exhale and slowly bend the knees toward the chest. The hips will incline upward. The knees should be in line with the hips in the tuck position. As you breathe, straighten your legs to resume the plank posture. Perform 1-3 sets of 5-10 repetitions.

Take Precautions

You should consult a doctor or physical therapist to determine the suitability of this exercise if you have a shoulder, neck, or back ailment. When performing this exercise, it is easy to hurt your shoulders, especially if you are using high weights or have bad form.

- Keep your exercises and motions slow and smooth.
- Steer clear of lifting bulky items.

- Work on maintaining excellent standing and sitting postures.

- Verify that the chair is strong and steady.

- Consume a healthy diet.

- Include protein in each meal.

- Eat seeds and nuts.

- Consume foods enriched with calcium.

- To find out which supplements to take, consult your doctor.

Advice

Your core strength declines with age, making even basic daily chores challenging. Exercise every day is the only method to maintain the health and strength of your core muscles. It might be difficult to carry out daily duties if one has weak core muscles, raising one's risk of falling, osteoporosis, and joint pain. Seniors should perform low-impact core exercises every day for 20 to 25 minutes. Examples include marching in place, marching with leg stretches, seated side bends, resistance band sidekicks, and laying ankle taps. Without causing any injury or aggravating any underlying issues, these exercises can significantly enhance your muscle tone and posture, agility, flexibility, and gait. The seated and laying workouts described here may be more appropriate for you if you suffer knee or back pain.

CHAPTER 4: ROUTINE EXERCISES

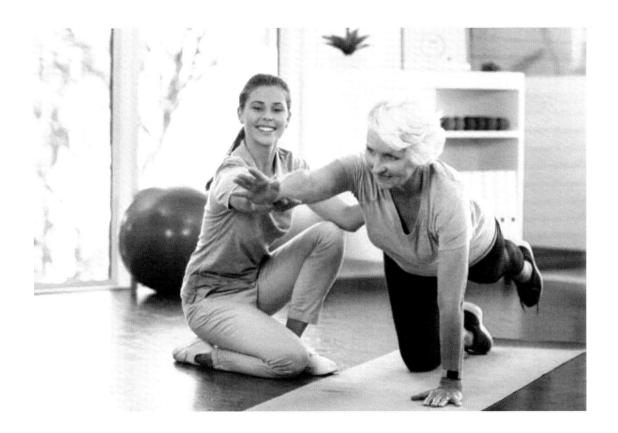

Level 1

If you are starting your core workout, this exercise routine can help you. Make sure to warm up well for 5-10 minutes before you start the workout.

Warm-Up
1. **Standing Crisscross crunches**: 10 Reps
2. **Back Rolls:** 2 minutes

Workout
1. **Seated Knee To-Chest**: 10 Reps
2. **Seated Forward Bends:** 10 Reps
3. **Lying Ankle Tap:** 30 seconds
4. **Wood Chops:** 10 Reps for each side
5. **Birddog:** 10 Reps for each side

Cool Down
1. **Cat/Cow:** 60 seconds
2. **Marching in place:** 2 minutes.

Note: As you progress each day, you can increase the frequency of each exercise by two reps.

Level 2

Only after following the level 1 routine for more than two weeks can you switch to this core exercise routine. Take 60-second gaps between each exercise to avoid excessive strain.

Warm-Up
1. **Standing Side Crunches**: 60 seconds
2. **Alternating Toe Touches:** 60 seconds

Workout
1. **March with Extended Legs**: 20 Reps
2. **Tummy Twists**: 10 Reps per side
3. **Leg Kicks:** 10 Reps for each leg
4. **Dead Bug:** 10 Reps
5. **Knee Planks**: 10 Reps
6. **Oblique Twists When Seated**: 10 Reps

Cool Down
1. **Standing Forward Bend**: 60 seconds

Note: make sure to use extra comfy quality yoga mats to try these exercises and keep your back straight while lying down during an exercise. If you have back pain issues, then consult your doctor first.

Level 3

This intermediate-advanced core exercise routine is created to strengthen the core muscle. Start with at least 5 minutes of warm-up before skipping to the workout.

Warm-Up
1. **Alternating Side Lunge**: 60 seconds
2. **Marching In Place**: 3 minutes

Workout
1. **Traditional Wood Chop**: 10 Reps per side
2. **Transferring a Core Ball**: 10 Reps
3. **Reverse Crunch**: 5 Reps per side
4. **Advanced Birddog:** 10 Reps
5. **Core Squats for Strength**: 10 Reps
6. **Extended Leg Raises**: 10 Reps

Cool Down
1. **Cat/Cow**: 60 seconds

Note: Breathe in and out consistently during each rep.

Level 4

Here comes the advanced combination of exercises that your core needs. Besides the suggested warm-up, you can also charge yourself with a 10-minute walk.

Warm-Up
1. **Standing Side Crunch:** 60 seconds
2. **Alternating Toe Touches:** 60 seconds
3. **Alternating Side Lunge:** 60 seconds

Workout
1. **Seated Side Bends:** 10 Reps per side
2. **Leg Raises:** 10 Reps per leg
3. **Advanced Birddog:** 10 Reps
4. **Twist with a Medicine Ball:** 10 Reps
5. **Dead Bug:** 10 Reps
6. **Core Squats for Strength:** 10 Reps

Cool Down
1. **Standing forward bend:** 60 seconds
2. **Marching In Place:** 2 minutes

Note: While doing the crunches, use your core muscles during the movement.

BOOK 4:
SENIOR RESISTANCE
BAND EXERCISES

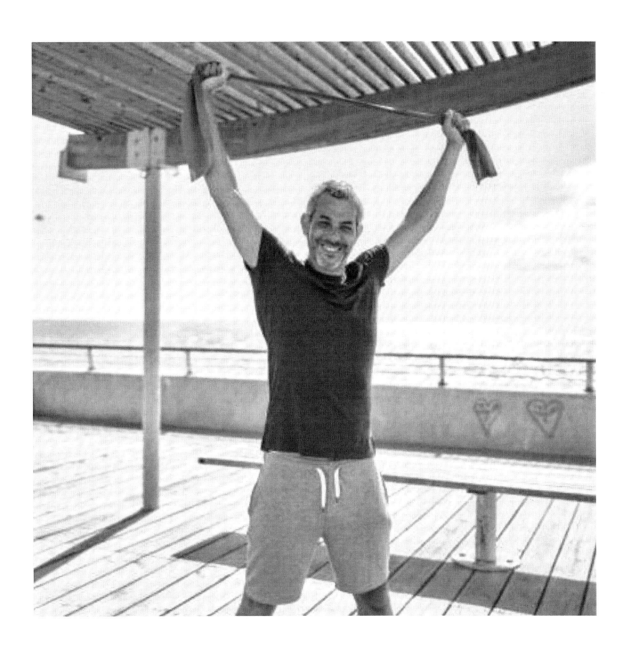

CHAPTER 1: RESISTANCE BAND WORKOUT

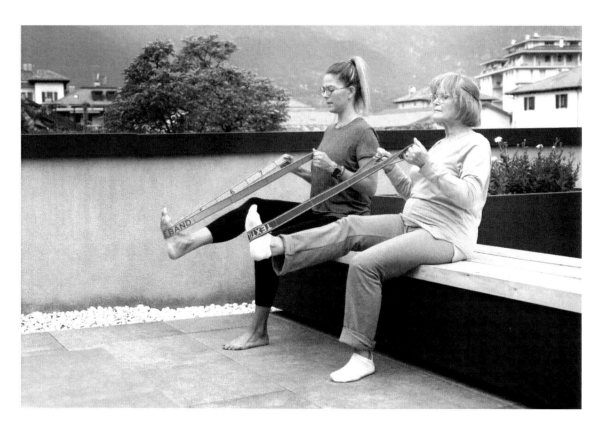

Resistance bands are excellent for people who like to work out at home or bring their exercises when they travel, but their benefits extend beyond these situations. This inexpensive exercise equipment has several advantages: ease, adaptability, safety, and efficacy. You'll be more inspired to incorporate resistance training into your home gym as you become more aware of its benefits.

Benefits of Resistance Band Workout

People of every age or fitness level can benefit from this affordable training equipment. But don't be fooled by their apparent simplicity. Exercises with resistance bands are surprisingly effective and have numerous advantages over conventional free weights. Here are just a few advantages that our professionals want you to be aware of:

An Efficient Exercise

Whether you buy them separately or as a set, resistance bands are an inexpensive addition to your home gym equipment. Even some bands include a DVD with exercise instructions.

Adapt Simply for Different Levels of Fitness

Various resistance levels exist for low, medium, or heavy bands. Simply adding or subtracting slack to the band during a workout will allow you to alter the resistance level. You may also combine many bands to heighten the difficulty.

Change Well-Known Exercises

Exercises with resistance bands usually borrow from well-known strength-training techniques. For instance, you can substitute the typical dumbbell bicep curl with this exercise: stand on one end of the cord, curl your arm up, and grasp the other.

Exercise Your Whole Body

Numerous kits provide suggested workouts for almost all of the body's major muscle groups. For instance, numerous exercises can be performed by stepping on a band's end or wrapping it around a stationary object.

Extend Storage Space Less

Resistance bands are an excellent option if you don't have much space for a home gym because they take up extraordinarily little area when not in use. After working out, you can coil them up, keep them in a box or drawer, or hang them on a hook.

Exercise on the Road

Resistance equipment is a terrific method to bring your workout with you when you travel because it is so small and portable. Numerous resistance band workouts are simple to perform in the cramped quarters of a hotel room.

Change Up Your Workouts

Your muscles get used to any new training routine over time. Cross-training using free weights, machines, and resistance band workouts is a smart idea to keep things interesting. Each will exercise your muscles a little bit differently.

Exercise Safely, Even When Alone

Resistance bands provide strength training without the chance of dumping a big weight on your foot or trapping your fingers between weight plates. They are, therefore, perfect for exercising when you don't have a personal trainer or workout buddy to guide you.

Get an Effective Workout

Both resistance bands and free weight exercises are efficient, despite certain distinctions. Think about the arc your arm forms when performing a bicep curl. The beginning of that arc is where free weights will feel the heaviest, while the arc's conclusion is where resistance bands will make your muscles work the hardest (when the band is most taut). Your muscles will work well because your body is moving against the opposition.

CHAPTER 2: TYPES OF RESISTANCE BANDS

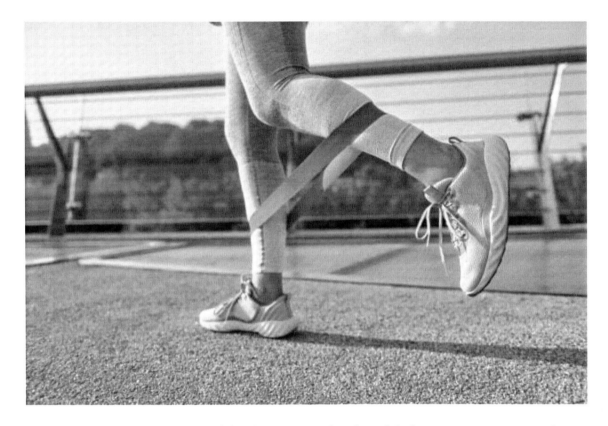

The famous latex or fabric loops (also known as tiny bands) that you wrap around your wrists, ankles, or thighs are a common component of resistance band exercises. But there are other band designs out there that are better suited for other exercises or motions. The main categories of resistance bands are described below.

Power Resistance Bands (AKA Loop Bands)

In essence, loop bands resemble enormous rubber bands. They are an endless flat loop that can serve several functions. Loop bands can be used for full-body workouts (squats, shoulder presses, thrusters, etc.), bodyweight assistance (pull-ups, dips, muscle ups, etc.), bodyweight resistance (pushups, bear crawls, box jumps), physical therapy (people with leg, back and knee injuries and help in recovery from torn MCL and ACL, knee replacement, patella, and meniscus rehab), warm-ups, static stretching (increased the stretch (squats with bands, bench press with bands, etc.). For pulling and pushing activities and rehabilitative exercises, you can secure them to a pole or bar (i.e., rotator cuff).

Power loop bands may be used for every area of training, whether athletic-focused or bodybuilder-oriented. They are incredibly adaptable, letting you work through all three planes of motion.

All power resistance bands have a thickness of 0.18 inches and a length of 41 inches. The band's width determines how the sizes differ. The amount of resistance depends on the width. The bands' widths range from 0.25 inches to 2.5 inches. So, if you had all the different sizes, your resistance would range from 5 to 175 pounds. Here are the bandwidths and resistance levels for SET as a reference:

- Yellow (1/2" thick): 5- 30 Pounds (41" x 0.5" x 0.18")

- Black (7/8" thick): 20 - 55 Pounds (41" x 0.85" x 0.18")

- Blue (1 1/4" thick): 35- 70 Pounds (41" x 1.25" x 0.18")

- Green (1 3/4" thick): 45 - 11 Pounds (41" x 1.75" x 0.18")

- Gray (2 1/2" thick): 60 - 170 Pounds (41" x 2.5" x 0.18")

Tube Resistance Bands with Handles

The handles on tube resistance bands are designed to resemble the handles on gym equipment like dumbbells. They quickly secure to a door or a bar or pole.

They benefit from chest presses, curls, back rows, shoulder presses, and other pressing and pulling workouts. Tube resistance bands are fantastic for people who don't have access to a gym or who prefer to train outside and want something basic and easily portable because they can work all of your muscle groups. Sets of tube bands typically provide 10 to 50 pounds of resistance. The resistance is dependent on the tube thickness.

Rubber Mini-Bands

Similar to Power Resistance Loop Bands but much shorter and wider are mini bands. For increased comfort and to prevent the band from rolling up, which frequently happens with noticeably light resistance small bands, new designs have fabrics covering the bands (we much prefer the non-slip fabric bands).

You can use little bands to strengthen and stabilize your lower body (and upper body with certain exercises).

You can achieve excellent hip and glute activation by positioning them slightly above your knees or at your ankles. They are beneficial to use when lifting weights. When performing movements like squats, hip thrusts, and leg extensions, mini bands can help you balance, activate your core, maintain good form, and get that activation and tension in the hips.

Like most resistance bands, tiny bands are an excellent instrument for stabilizing the shoulder and elbow joints and can effectively address shoulder complexes. Mini bands can help you prepare for actions like handstands and muscle-ups if you enjoy calisthenics.

Mini-band sets are typically described as either light, medium, heavy, or extra heavy. This should be 5 to 50 pounds or more of resistance. Depending on their resistance, these bands will range in length and thickness, but they are all designed to be wrapped around the legs.

Light Therapy Resistance Bands

Therapy bands are thin, light 'free bands,' which do not loop and are exceptionally long (up to 7 feet) (although you could tie them in a knot to create a loop). Therapy bands are designed for older persons who desire a very low-impact workout as well as people who are recovering their strength from an accident.

They perform well with Pilates exercises and fat-burning routines since you only need a little extra resistance to feel the burn. This is how many ladies utilize light therapy bands to tone their muscles. They can also be used for dynamic stretching during warm-ups and static stretching at the end of a workout. These bands can assist you in extending your stretch and enhancing your mobility and range of motion. Therapy band sets typically give 3–10 pounds of resistance.

Figure 8 Bands

The shape of Figure 8 bands is exactly what the name implies. They have soft handles at the top and bottom of the figure-8 shape. They can be stretched as far as necessary to target your upper and lower bodies. Figure 8 bands can be used for lateral movements similar to mini bands and for exercises resembling machine and dumbbell exercises to tube resistance bands. In the sagittal and lateral planes of motion, pushing and pulling workouts benefit most from their utilization. Figure 8 band setups will typically provide 8–20 pounds of resistance.

Factors to Consider Before Buying Resistance Bands

Purchase a Range of Bands

The strength or tension of the band is the main factor to consider when purchasing a resistance band. If you're just starting, pick a light band. Bands are usually color-coded, with yellow for light and black for heavy, to assist you in deciding what to pick. However, remember that many brands and goods use different color schemes. It is recommended to look for a kit with three to five resistance levels. As you gain stronger, they provide e a solid spectrum for diverse activities and leave room for progress.

Place Quality First

When making your purchase, you should also search for high-quality bands. I advise against using a resistance band that will become sticky or break in the middle of a workout. A thicker band will typically be stronger. Before each workout, it's a good idea to check the band and rubber for signs of wear and tear; if you find any cracks or damage, it's time to replace the item.

Consider the Material Type

You can purchase resistance bands composed of elastic fabric or rubber latex. We prefer fabric loops over latex since they are more pleasant and durable. Additionally, fabric bands don't slide or roll up when you're working out. Fabric bands are, therefore, often the best choice for lower body exercises. Latex bands may provide more stretch for stretching, joint stability exercises, explosive motions, and upper body exercises. Using resistance bands safely will help you prevent being hurt.

CHAPTER 3: EXERCISES TO WARM UP AND COOL DOWN

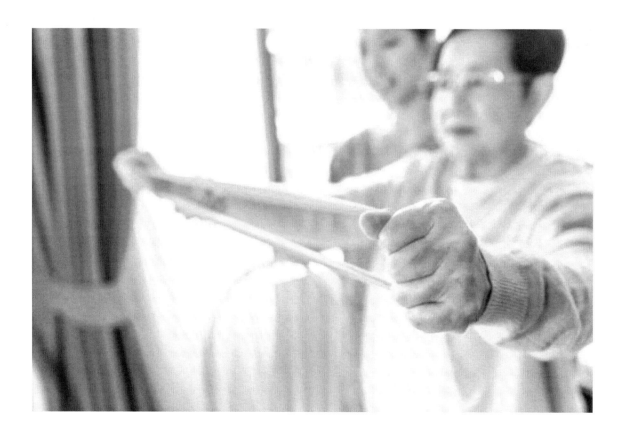

Shoulder Circles

Shoulder circles are a resistance band warm-up workout. Pulling your shoulders back and down will help you stand tall. Take two light resistance bands, lock the end of the elastic bands under each foot and pull them with your hands. Stretch your arms out to the sides while holding an exercise band in each hand. Try to maintain strain on the resistance band and make small circles with your shoulders by rotating them clockwise and then counterclockwise

Face Pulls

Face pulls are a resistance band warm-up workout. The workout band should be securely fastened to a surface near your face. Take hold of the elastic band with both hands and move backward a few feet. Stretch your arms before you while applying light resistance to the resistance band. Pull your hands up to your face at this point. Ensure that your elbows are raised. After a brief period of holding this position, go back to your beginning position.

Standing Crunch

Keep your feet hip-width apart and your core engaged. Holding your band with hands in front of your chest with your arms outstretched at shoulder height. Lift your left leg and press it toward your right hand while keeping your arms out. Immediately after putting your left foot back on the ground, thrust your right knee toward your left hand. Reset your right foot on the ground. Alternate the sides as you continue this pattern.

Side Stretch

Stand tall with your hands on your hips, your elbows bent, and your feet slightly wider than hip distance apart. This is where everything begins. Reach your left arm up and over your body while bending your torso to the right, keeping your right hand on your right hip. To get back to the beginning position, reverse the motion. On the opposite side, repeat. Alternate the sides as you continue this pattern.

Jab

With your torso tilted, take a staggered stance with your left foot in front of your right. Divide your weight on the balls of your feet and gently bend your knees. Your hands should be in fists, your elbows should be bent, and your hands should be held just below your chin.

Your left arm should be extended while your legs are slightly bouncing. Pull your left arm back to chin level swiftly. Without pausing, turn your torso slightly to the left while extending your right arm. Bring your right arm back quickly to chin level. Continually throw punches in this pattern.

Squat to Row

With your feet hip-width apart and your core engaged, stand tall. Hold the band with both arms before your chest after folding it in half. Send your hips back and squat by bending your knees to at least 90 degrees as you do so. Maintain a long arm position. Standing up, complete a row by pulling your shoulder blades together to pull the band toward your chest to get back to the beginning position. Your elbows will extend and flare backward. At the top, squeeze your glutes. To turn the row around, pause, then straighten your elbows. Squat down again right away to continue the pattern.

Seated Static Hold

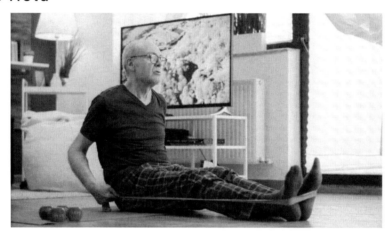

Pulling your shoulder blades together while still seated, push the band toward your chest with your hands facing each other. Your elbows have to be spread wide to the sides and remember to keep your back straight. Maintain the posture as in the image above fore 5-10 seconds.

Upward-Facing Dog

Lie face down on a mat and assume a low cobra position by elevating your chest with

your hands and bending at the lower back. With your elbows slightly bent, support the body's weight on your hands.

Lying Torso Twist

Lie on your back and bring your knees in towards your chest. With your shoulder blades square onto the floor and your arms stretched out so you're in a T shape, move your knees down to one side. Look in the opposite direction to your legs and hold. Return to the center and repeat the stretch on the other side. This exercise is perfect to stretch the back and the abdominal part.

Neck Circles

Stand tall and with your feet shoulder-width apart. Move your neck in circles, first clockwise and then anti-clockwise.

Kneeling Shin Quad Stretch

Your quads and shins will be stretched with this easy exercise. Perform this after your cool-down. Slowly sit down on your legs, starting from a kneeling position while maintaining the tops of your feet on the ground and remember to keep your back straight. After maintaining this stance for 20–30 seconds, release.

CHAPTER 4: RESISTANCE BAND EXERCISES

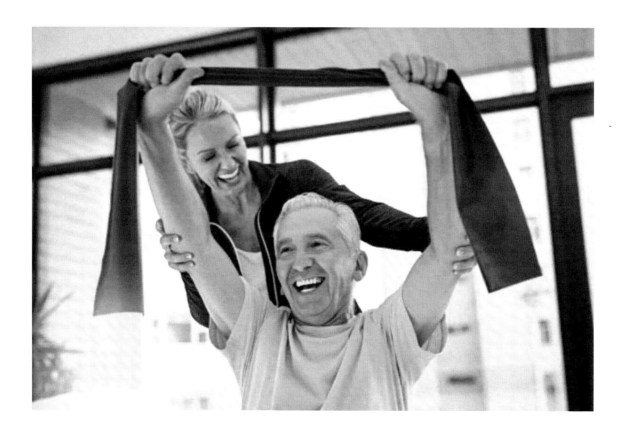

Beginner and Intermediate Level

Kicks

Kicks are a resistance band warm-up activity. For this exercise, you'll need a short-loop resistance band. Position the band at the height of your quads by stepping into it with both feet (just above the knees). Swing your right leg slowly and deliberately forth and back. Do this exercise once more using your left leg.

The Marching Hip Bend (Seated)

For this exercise, you'll need a short-loop resistance band. Position the band at the height of your quads by stepping into it with both feet (just above the knees). While you are seated on a chair, stretch the band by lifting one knee toward the chest. Hold for five seconds, then slowly return to the ground. Up to 15 times, then switch legs. Observe your breathing and remember to keep your back straight.

Side Bend

Stand tall and with your feet shoulder-width apart. Hold the resistance band firmly between your palms while raising your arms above your head. Alternate between bending your upper body to the left and right sides.

Shovel Workout (Seated)

Sit shoulder-width apart on a chair with your feet flat on the floor. Wrap a band around one foot's bottom. Breathe easily, engage your core, and keep your posture upright.

Hold the band's ends firmly in both palms at hip height. Slowly bend the knee towards the chest while maintaining a high arch. To straighten the knee, lower the foot toward the ground. Up to 15 times, then switch legs. Focus on your breathing.

Flexing the Shoulders (Seated)

Set up and beginning position: place your shoulders apart while sitting on a chair with your feet on the floor. Hold the band tightly in both hands and loop it under the knees. To maintain proper posture, let your shoulders down, and your core tighten. Pull the band as high as it is comfortable for you while holding your right arm straight and your thumb up. Five seconds of holding the band up. Return to the starting position gradually. Up to 15 times, then switch arms. Observe your breathing

External Rotation of the Shoulder (Band Pull Apart)

Keep your feet flat, place them on the ground, and sit up straight in a chair. Hold the band firmly in both hands, shoulder-width apart, elbows bent at your sides, and thumbs facing up. Breathe, engage your core, keep your posture upright and extend both arms forward.

Hold the band while keeping the position for 5 seconds. Return hands to starting position slowly. Up to 15 times. Observe your breathing. During this moment, relax your body and mind.

Ankle Pumps

Stand with a straight back and take hold of the band's ends with both hands. Wrap the band around your foot's ball. Apply pressure to the band with your foot like you would a gas pedal. Return to the starting position. Repeat with the opposite leg, 10 times.

Clamshell

Place your feet close together on the bed while bending your knees. Tie a band around your legs slightly above your knees. Starting with your legs together, try to spread your legs as far as you can. Slowly return to the beginning position.

Seated Clamshell

Tie the band around your legs just above the knees in the first position. Push your legs to the side while keeping your ankles tucked in, then slowly return to the starting position. Up to 10 times.

Hamstring Curls

Fasten the band to the leg of a chair in front of you. Wrap the band around your ankle and, with your hands on the back of the chair, bend the knee and draw your heel back in the opposite direction to the chair. Retrace your steps to the beginning place. On the opposite side, repeat.

Seated Leg Press

Bend your knee and loop the band under the middle of your foot while holding the ends of the band in each hand. Push your leg straight out and down against the band while maintaining your elbows at your sides. Retrace your steps to the beginning place. Repeat with the other leg and remember to keep your back straight.

Sitting Ankle Press

While sitting on a chair with a straight back, take hold of a band end in each hand. Wrap the band around your foot's ball. Apply pressure to the band with your foot like you would a gas pedal. Repeat with the opposite leg.

Forward Kick

Stand with your back to the door and put one of your legs through the band's loop. Fasten the end of the band securely to the bottom of the door and step forward with your leg to pull the band. Go back to the beginning position gradually. On the opposite side, repeat.

Backward Kick

Stand in front of the door with one of your legs in the loop of the band. Fasten the end of the band securely to the bottom of the door. Move your leg back while keeping your body straight. Go back to the beginning position gradually. On the opposite side, repeat.

Kick Out to the Side

Stand facing the door with your side up. Place the band on the ankle that is furthest from the entrance. Move a little bit away from the door to make the band tighter. Extend your leg away from the door while maintaining a forward toe. Retrace your steps to the beginning point. On the opposite side, repeat.

Stand with Your Side Towards the Entrance

Place the band on the ankle that is closest to the door. Move a few inches away from the door to squeeze the band tighter. Step aside from the door by crossing your leg over your torso. Keep your toes always pointed forward. Retrace your steps to the beginning point. On the opposite side, repeat.

Resisting Side-Stepping

Tie the band around your legs slightly above the knees. Start by spreading your legs out to shoulder width. Slightly squat down by bending slightly at the waist and knees. While taking a step to the side, maintain this posture. Return to the beginning position gradually while maintaining a tight band. Step over to the opposite side and repeat.

Sit Straight Up

With your legs shoulder-width apart, loop the band under your feet and hold the band with your hands. While you are sitting, stand up while maintaining a firm grasp on the band and your elbows at your sides. Remember to keep your back straight as you stand up. Retrace to the beginning point.

Arm Curls

With your arms shoulder-width apart, grasp one end of the band in each hand. Place both your hands in your lap. While the band is kept in your lap with one hand, bring the other hand close to your chest by bending the opposite arm at the elbow. On the opposite side, repeat.

Arm Raise

Hold one end of the band in each hand. Begin by positioning both of your hands in front of your left leg. You keep your left hand away from your thigh. Put your right hand over your right shoulder and extend your right arm up and across your body. Retrace your steps to the beginning point. Continue by using your other arm.

Chest Press

Hold a band end in each hand as you press your chest. Place the band below your armpits and wrap it over your upper back. Maintain a relaxed, at-your-side position with your elbows bent. Squeeze the band with your arms extended straight out. Return to the starting position gradually.

Arm Extension

Hold one end of the band in each hand, shoulder-width apart. Put both of your hands on your chest. While the other arm extends straight to your lap, the first arm retains the band against your chest. Go back to the beginning position gradually. Continue by using your other arm. Holding one end of the band in each hand, perform shoulder blade squeezes. Maintain a natural elbow bend at chest height. Pull your elbows back while squeezing your shoulder blades together. Retrace your steps to the beginning point.

Bicep Curls

Keep your feet above your resistance band. Take hold of both ends with both hands. Raise your arms to the level of your chest and keep a 90-degree angle of your arms for 5 seconds. Remember to keep your back straight while you are doing this exercise. Repeat ten to fifteen times. This can be carried out either by sitting down or standing up.

Sitting Row

Place your feet flat on the ground and sit up straight in a chair. Hold the band tightly in both hands and loop it under one foot. Breathe, engage your core, and keep your posture upright. To perform a seated row, squeeze your shoulder blades together and push your elbow straight back until your hands are at the top of your hips. After holding for five seconds, carefully return to the starting position. Always keep your arms by your side. Up to 15 times, repeat (switch arms). Keep breathing.

Raising the Toe and Heel (Seated)

Put both of your feet inside the loop of a loop band, then wrap the band over your thighs Lift both toes off the ground while pressing the sides of your thighs against the band. Avoid allowing the band to pull your knees or ankles inward. Hold for 5 seconds, then take your position at the beginning. Lift your heels off the ground. Up to 15 times, repeat. Observe your breathing.

Sidewalk

Sidewalks are a good place to start a resistance band warmup. For this exercise, you'll need a short resistance band. Put both of your feet inside the loop of a loop band, then wrap the band over your thighs. Hold your hands in front of your body while bending your knees and facing forward with your upper body. Move to the side one step. Throughout the entire maneuver, the band should be under tension. Perform the workout both ways.

Deadlift

Your feet should be hip width apart on the resistance band as it is laid on the ground. Take the exercise band in your hands with both ends grasped. Maintain a straight back. Get up and stand up by lifting your hips and knees. As you rise, tense your glutes. Return to a position when your hands are at shin height.

Advanced Level

Squat Hip

Set up and beginning position: place your shoulders apart while sitting on a chair with your feet on the floor. Just above the knee, wrap the band around your thighs, then tie it on top. Breathe easily, engage your core, and keep your posture upright. To release the band, push out the thighs and hold for three to five seconds. Return to the starting position slowly. Relax, then do it fifteen times. Observe your breathing.

Squat Knee Flexion

Setup and position at the outset: Sit shoulder-width apart on a chair with your feet flat on the floor. Just above the shoes, wrap the band around the ankles and fasten it. Breathe easily, engage your core, and keep your posture upright.

Bench Press

Place your feet flat on the ground and sit up straight in a chair. Hold the band tightly in both hands and loop it behind your back. To maintain proper posture, let your shoulders down, and your core tighten. Grasp the ends of the band with your thumbs facing up. Elbows firmly at your sides. Starting with your hands near your chest, try to extend both arms forward and keep this position for 5 seconds. Up to 15 repetitions, remember to observe your breathing.

Other Exercises with Resistance Band

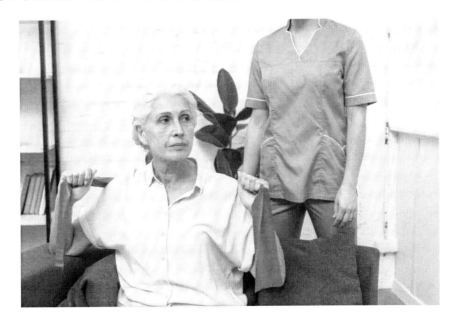

Place your back straight and your abs tense while sitting in a firm chair. Take hold of the resistance band's two ends. Your elbows should be bent and in front of your chest in this position. You can fold your resistance band in half if it is too lengthy before beginning. As you exhale, draw the band closer to your chest while attempting to straighten your arms. Breathe in and exhale. Repeat 10 to 15 times after returning to your starting position. You can perform this exercise either seated or standing.

Lateral Raise

Step on the center of the resistance band with both feet flat on the ground. Take hold of your band's grips. Return to the starting position after raising both arms to shoulder height on the side. Repeat ten to fifteen times.

Squats

Step on the center of the resistance band with both feet flat on the ground.

Take hold of the band's two ends. Slowly stoop down by bending your knees. Your knees should be behind your toes, and your butt should be out. Go back to the beginning position. Repeat ten to fifteen times.

Chest Press

Place the resistance band behind your shoulders while holding onto both ends. Return to the beginning posture by extending both arms in front of your chest. Repeat ten to fifteen times. This exercise can be performed either seated or standing.

Leg Press

Place your back straight in a firm chair. Take hold of the resistance band at both ends. Center your band around your right foot. Keep the left foot flat on the ground. Straighten the right leg out in front of you. Get back into a position where you started. With each leg, repeat between 10 and 15 times.

Triceps Press

Keep the resistance band under your right heel while you are standing. Stretch the opposite end of the band so that you are holding both ends behind your right ear. Pull it back behind your ears after releasing it above your head. Repeat on each side 10 to 15 times.

Calf

Put your right foot in the center of the band and press one while sitting upright in a firm chair. Use your hands to hold both ends. Stretch your right leg before you and point your toes at the ceiling. After that, flex your toes and look down. Repeat on each side 10 to 15 times.

Bent Over Row

Joint issues, especially those in your hips, will be relieved by this excellent workout. Pay close attention to maintaining good back support throughout the activity.

Place a chair so that your back is well-supported. Hold the resistance band firmly beneath your feet while holding onto both ends with your hands. Keep your back straight as you bend until your body is almost parallel to the ground. With your elbows elevated and your arms raised so they are parallel to your shoulders, lift the resistance band with your arms as many times as you feel comfortable, lower your arms once more and repeat.

Hip Abduction

You may improve your hip rotations, bolster your hip muscles, and lessen joint pain by performing hip abductions daily. Sit down and make sure your back is well-supported. Keep your legs parallel to the ground. Above your knees, wrap the resistance band. To move your knees in oppositional directions, use your hips. Repeat the exercise by bringing your knees back to the middle.

Hip Extension

You may focus on developing healthy hips by including hip extensions in your workout. Hip extensions can be carried out while standing or, for a change, while seated. Take your resistance band and wrap one ankle with it. One end should be wrapped around solid support. You can support yourself by holding onto the back of the chair and using a chair leg. Lift your leg as far back as you can or straight behind you. Put your leg back in its original position. Before switching legs, repeat.

How to Prepare for Resistance Band Exercises

Experts suggest warming your body up with a quick, vigorous walk before practice. Try active stretches, including lunges, squats, and arm circles. These inform your body that it will be exercising. Before beginning to exert more significant strain on your muscles with specific workouts, the objective is to encourage your muscles to feel loose.

Starting each session with a few minutes of balancing training is also important. This could involve putting one leg up to hip height and holding it while standing tall next to a table (hanging onto it if necessary). Alternatively, you can adopt a wide stance while slowly moving to one side while elevating the foot to the other.

Balance training can assist you in maintaining safe movement patterns during resistance training while enhancing daily function. Exercises that promote balance also increase the safety of your workout by teaching your neuromuscular system to maintain balance throughout each movement.

CHAPTER 5: ROUTINE EXERCISES

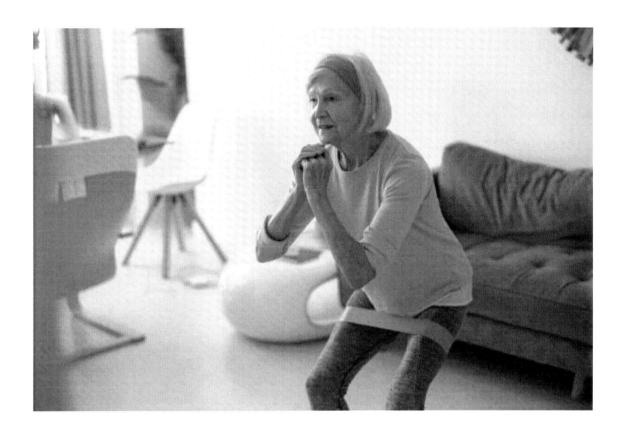

Routine 1

Use the light therapy resistance bands to carry out this exercise routine. First, practice stretching the bands 2-3 times to get used to it, and then start following this routine.

Warm-Up

1. **Standing Crunch:** 60 seconds
2. **Side Stretch:** 60 seconds
3. **Kneeling Shin Quad Stretch:** 60 seconds

Workout

1. **Side Bend:** 10 reps on each side
2. **Forward Kick:** 10 reps each leg
3. **Arm Curls:** 10 reps per side
4. **Lateral Raise:** 10 Reps
5. **Squats:** 10 Reps
6. **Chest Press:** 10 Reps
7. **Hip extension:** 10 Reps
8. **Squat Hip:** 10 Reps
9. **Bench Press:** 10 Reps

Cool Down

1. **Neck Circles:** 60 seconds
2. **Lying Torso Twist:** 60 seconds

Note: Do not overextend your joints while doing any of the given exercises.

Routine 2

Try to keep the tension on the muscles and not the bones while using the resistance bands. The resistance band might snap back into its original form if your joints don't secure.

Warm-Up

1. **Jab:** 60 seconds
2. **Squat to Row:** 60 seconds
3. **Seated Static Hold:** 60 seconds

Workout

1. **Sitting Row:** 10 Reps
2. **Bicep Curls:** 10 Reps on each side
3. **Chest Press:** 10 Reps
4. **Sidewalk:** 2 minutes
5. **Bent Over Row:** 10 Reps
6. **Calf:** 10 Reps

Cool Down

1. **Kneeling Shin Quad Stretch:** 60 seconds
2. **Standing Crunch:** 60 seconds

Note: Perform the resistance band stretches in a slow and controlled manner. You don't have to fight the bands to stretch them, slowly move your body parts to make the stretch.

Routine 3

While training with this resistance band routine, deep breathing is the most important thing you should not forget. It empowers you to do each rep.

Warm-Up

1. **Upward-Facing Dog**: 60 seconds
2. **Lying Torso Twist**: 60 seconds

Workout

1. **The Marching Hip Bend (Seated)**: 10 Reps
2. **Raising the Toe and Heel (Seated)**: 10 Reps
3. **Backward Kick:** 10 Reps
4. **Ankle Pumps**: 10 Reps
5. **Shovel Workout (Seated)**: 10 Reps
6. **Hamstring Curls**: 10 Reps

Cool Down

1. **Neck Circles:** 60 seconds
2. **Shoulder Circles:** 60 seconds

Note: Resistance band training is comparatively more difficult than the core and stretching exercises I have explained in previous sections. So, if you are a beginner, I would advise you to start with non-band exercises and gradually introduce resistance band exercises.

BOOK 5:
ARTHRITIS EXERCISES
FOR SENIORS

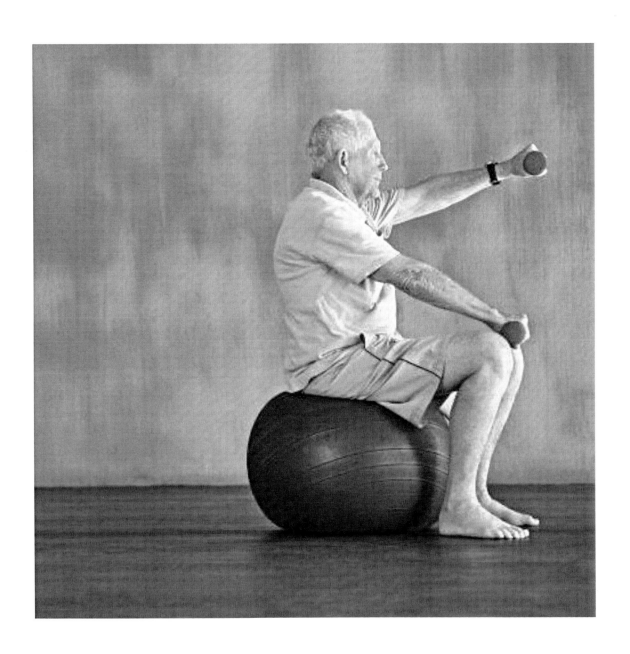

CHAPTER 1: INTRODUCTION TO ARTHRITIS

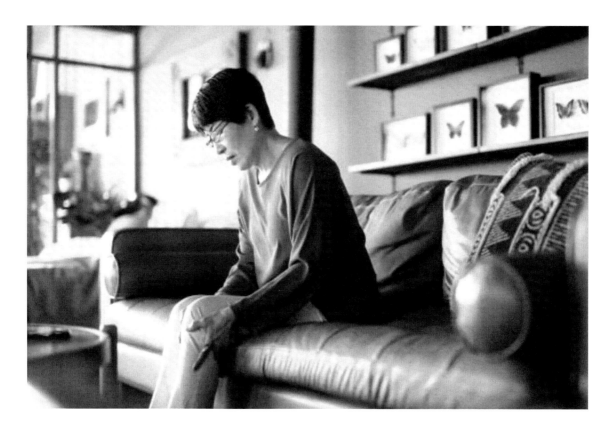

Over 100 disorders fall under the umbrella category of arthritis. "Arthritis" literally translates to "joint inflammation." One of your body's natural responses to illness or damage is inflammation. Swelling, discomfort, and stiffness are all part of it. Tissue damage can result from inflammation that lasts long or keeps coming back, as in arthritis. A joint, such as the hip or knee joint, is where two or more bones meet. Your joints' bones are coated with cartilage, a supple, smooth substance. It protects your bones and makes it painless for the joint to move.

The synovium lines the joint. The synovium's lining creates synovial fluid, a lubricant that hydrates the joint and reduces internal friction. The joint capsule is a robust fibrous covering that surrounds it. Ligaments are sturdy tissue bands that link the bones and support the joint's stability. Your joints are supported and moved by your muscles and tendons.

When a joint or the area around it gets inflamed, arthritis results, causing discomfort, stiffness, and occasionally trouble moving. Some arthritis can also affect the skin, internal organs, and other body parts. One in five adults suffers from arthritis. Anyone can experience it, but as you become older, it happens more frequently.

Types of Arthritis

Osteoarthritis

The most typical kind is this. Your bones' ends' cartilage starts to erode as a result. The bones start to collide as a result. Your fingers, knees, or hips could all hurt. Osteoarthritis causes cartilage to degenerate, which usually occurs as people age. Because of this, osteoarthritis is occasionally referred to as a degenerative joint disease. However, if there are additional factors, it may start much earlier. For instance, a fracture close to a joint or an athletic injury like a torn anterior cruciate ligament (ACL) can result in arthritis. It can affect any joint, but the hands and weight-bearing joints, including the knee, hip, and facet joints (in particular), are most usually affected.

Arthritis Rheumatica

This chronic condition can impact any joint, although the hands, wrists, and knees are the most usually affected areas. The immune system, which serves as the body's defense against infection, wrongly assaults the joints in rheumatoid arthritis, resulting in swelling of the joint lining. Inflammation can harm bone and cartilage when it spreads to adjacent tissues. Rheumatoid arthritis can, in more severe forms, affect the skin, eyes, nerves, and other bodily organs.

Gout

This painful ailment develops when the body can't get rid of uric acid, a chemical that occurs naturally. In the joints, the extra uric acid crystallizes into needle-like structures that cause acute pain, swelling, and inflammation.

What Causes Arthritis?

Numerous forms of arthritis lack an identified etiology. Researchers are investigating how lifestyle and genetics (heredity) interact to cause arthritis. Your risk of developing arthritis may increase due to several factors, such as:

- **Age:** Your joints tend to deteriorate over time. Age increases the likelihood of having arthritis, particularly osteoarthritis.

- **Sex:** Besides gout, women are more likely to develop arthritis.

- **Genes:** Some forms of arthritis are hereditary. Some diseases, like lupus, ankylosing spondylitis, and rheumatoid arthritis, are correlated with specific genes.

- **Extra weight:** Obesity increases wear and strain on weight-bearing joints and raise the risk of arthritis, particularly osteoarthritis.

- **Injuries:** They may harm joints, leading to some forms of the disorder.

- **Infection:** Inflammation in the joints can be brought on by bacterial, viral, or fungal infections.

- **Work.** Some jobs requiring heavy lifting or repetitive motions can stress the joints or injure them, resulting in arthritis, especially osteoarthritis. For example, you may be more prone to developing osteoarthritis if your job usually requires bending and squatting your knees.

Symptoms

The symptoms of various forms of arthritis might vary in severity from person to person. In most cases, osteoarthritis does not manifest symptoms outside of the joint. Fatigue, a fever, a rash, and joint inflammation indicate different types of arthritis.

- Pain
- Swelling
- Stiffness

- Tenderness
- Redness
- Warmth
- Joint deformity

In What Way is Arthritis Diagnosed?

The first step in treatment is a diagnosis of arthritis. Your doctor will: Consider your entire medical background. This will describe your symptoms as well.

- **Examine Your Health.** Your doctor will examine your joints for swelling, soreness, redness, warmth, or loss of motion.

- **Employ Imaging Tests, such as X-rays.** These can usually identify the type of arthritis you have. Osteoarthritis is diagnosed via X-rays, which usually reveal bone spurs, a lack of cartilage, and bone rubbing on bone in extreme cases.

- **Check the Joint Fluid.** Blood tests and joint aspiration are occasionally employed to distinguish osteoarthritis from other forms.

  Testing body fluids typically determine the diagnosis and course of treatment for the affected joint if your doctor considers infectious arthritis a consequence of another illness.

- **Test Your Pee or Blood.** These examinations can assist in identifying the type of arthritis you have or help your doctor rule out other conditions as the source of your symptoms.

  Rheumatoid factors (RF), antibodies that most persons with rheumatoid arthritis have in their blood but may also be present in other conditions, are detected in blood testing for rheumatoid arthritis.

- **The Anti-CCP Test.** This is a recent test for rheumatoid arthritis, which examines antibody levels in the blood. It is more accurate and likely to be higher only in patients who have or are about to develop rheumatoid arthritis. Anti-CCP antibodies may also identify those developing more severe cases of rheumatoid arthritis.

CHAPTER 2: MANAGEMENT OF ARTHRITIS

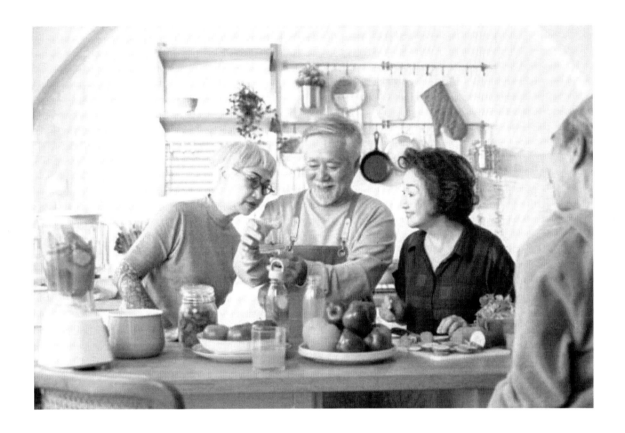

Eating the Right Food

It is real. Several meals can assist in reducing the symptoms of arthritis and enhance your overall joint health. A healthy diet can reduce inflammatory responses from the body that produce pain in addition to the usage of drugs. Eating the correct meals also aids in maintaining a healthy weight, which is crucial because your hips and knees support the majority, if not all, of your body weight. Try the following foods to reduce the discomfort from your arthritis:

Fish

Salmon, mackerel, and tuna are rich sources of vitamin D and Omega-3 fatty acids. These two have been shown to aid in reducing inflammation. We advise consuming fish once or twice every week as part of a healthy diet. Fish oil pills are an option for people who don't consume fish.

Dark Greens Leafy

Vitamins E and C are abundant in kale, broccoli, collard greens, spinach, and other vegetables. The body is defended by vitamin E from inflammatory chemicals. Collagen, a crucial component of cartilage that promotes joint flexibility, is made by the body with the assistance of vitamin C.

Nuts

Nuts, including almonds, hazelnuts, peanuts, pecans, pistachios, and walnuts, are rich in fiber, calcium, magnesium, zinc, vitamin E, and omega-3 fatty acids, all of which have anti-inflammatory properties. Additionally, nuts are heart-healthy, which is crucial for persons with rheumatoid arthritis (RA), who have a twice-as-high risk of developing heart disease as healthy adults.

Avocado Oil

Heart-healthy lipids are abundant in extra virgin olive oil, which also contains oleocanthal, a substance resembling non-steroidal anti-inflammatory medicines' effects. It has also been demonstrated that vitamin D and olive oil together can prevent bone loss.

Berries

Berries include two different anti-inflammatory compounds. Antioxidants, which are found in abundance in all fruits, can help combat inflammation. Additionally, anthocyanins, which lessen inflammation, are present in foods including blueberries, raspberries, strawberries, and blackberries.

Onions and Garlic

Unbelievably, these spicy vegetables contain anti-inflammatory compounds that have been demonstrated to reduce the discomfort associated with some types of arthritis. Additionally, they have the added benefit of enhancing immunity.

Leaf tea

Epigallocatechin-3-gallate is a type of natural antioxidant in this moderate beverage (EGCG). It has been demonstrated that this substance inhibits the body's generation of some inflammatory molecules, particularly those linked to arthritis. Additionally, recent research suggests that EGCG may delay cartilage aging, prolonging the lifespan of joints.

While it's vital to include as many foods as mentioned earlier in your diet as possible, there are several that you should aim to avoid. Red meat, fried foods, and packaged baked goods are high in saturated and trans fats. These foods are generally unhealthy and can result in weight gain, which can exacerbate symptoms.

Aloe Vera

Aloe vera is usually employed in complementary medicine. It comes in various forms, like pills, powder, gel, and leaves. Aloe vera is usually used to treat minor skin irritations like sunburn, but it can also ease joint pain. Nonsteroidal anti-inflammatory medicines (NSAIDs), usually used to treat arthritic pain, have anti-inflammatory qualities, are generally well tolerated, and don't have any adverse gastrointestinal side effects. A gel may be applied straight to the skin. In 2014, several researchers hypothesized that ingesting aloe could lessen the discomfort of osteoarthritis. To establish the effectiveness of these medicines, additional research is required. Aloe vera use is probably safe, according to the National Center for Complementary and Integrative Health (NCCIH); however, some persons taking it orally may experience negative effects. It could decrease blood glucose levels and interfere with some diabetes drugs.

Eucalyptus

People utilize eucalyptus as a readily available treatment for a variety of ailments. Eucalyptus leaf extracts are used in topical treatments for arthritis pain. The plant's leaves contain tannins, which may be useful in easing arthritis-related pain and swelling. Heat pads are sometimes used as a follow-up to maximize the results. Eucalyptus essential oils may lessen the symptoms of arthritis rheumatica.

Before using, always dilute an essential oil with carrier oil. Use two tablespoons of almond or any neutral oil and 15 drops of oil. Before applying topical eucalyptus, be cautious about conducting a patch test to check for allergies. On your forearm, apply a tiny amount of the product. It should be safe if there is no reaction within 24 to 48 hours.

Ginger

Although ginger is usually used in cooking, it may also offer health advantages. According to 2016 research, the same substances that give ginger its potent flavor also have anti-inflammatory benefits. According to some studies, ginger may one day replace NSAIDs. Ginger has long been used to relieve nausea in traditional medicine, but it can also treat arthritis rheumatica, osteoarthritis and joint and muscular pain.

In the future, components of ginger may serve as the foundation of pharmacological treatment for rheumatoid arthritis. It might not only aid in symptom management but also in preventing bone deterioration. Ginger can be consumed in several ways. These may consist of the following:

- Add powdered ginger to baked goods and prepare tea by steeping tea bags or fresh ginger in hot water for five minutes.
- Incorporating fresh or powdered ginger root into savory meals.
- Sprinkling a salad or stir dish with grated fresh ginger.

The number of active components in a cup of ginger tea may or may not aid with symptom relief. Ginger consumption in food and beverages can be much lower than in oral supplements. You can discuss ginger supplements and the dosage required to experience a therapeutic impact with a doctor.

CHAPTER 3: HOW EXERCISE HELPS PEOPLE WITH ARTHRITIS

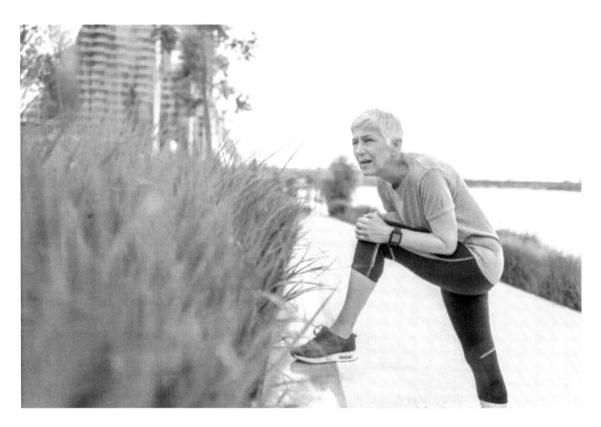

Your health and fitness can be improved through exercise without endangering your joints. Exercise can help with your current treatment plan since it:

- Consolidate the muscles that surround your joints.

- Assist you in maintaining bone density

- Give you extra vigor to go through the day, make it simpler to get a restful night's sleep, aid in weight management

- Improve the quality of your life

- Become more balanced

Despite what you might believe, exercise won't worsen your joint pain and stiffness. Your joints can become even more painful and stiff from inactivity. That's because maintaining the strength of your muscles and supporting tissue is essential to sustaining bone support. Lack of exercise causes those supporting muscles to deteriorate, which puts a greater strain on your joints.

Warm-Up and Cool-Down Exercises

People with arthritis need to exercise. It improves stamina and flexibility, eases joint discomfort, and lessens weariness. Of course, walking around the block or swimming a few lengths may seem overwhelming when stiff and sore joints are already making you feel exhausted. However, you don't have to be an Olympic swimmer or run a marathon to be able to aid with arthritic symptoms. Even light exercise helps you maintain a healthy weight and can reduce your pain. Exercise keeps you mobile even when arthritis threatens to render you immobile.

Sit Stand

Include this full-body muscle-strengthening workout in your home fitness regimen since maintaining muscular strength helps support joints. You can carry it out indoors or in your backyard. Start by doing this. Place your feet flat on the ground, knees aligned, and sit in a firm chair or bench. Press your heels down and stand while maintaining a straight back and forward-facing arms. Sit down slowly by bending your knees and hips while standing on your heels. 8 to 12 times total.

Leg Figure Eights

Sit with your knees bent and your legs in front of you. Raise your feet together while holding the edge of a sturdy chair or bench. Tighten your abs. For 30 to 60 seconds, perform tight figure eights in the air.

Standing Pushups

Stand with your feet hip-width apart a few feet away, facing a wall, behind a robust outdoor bench, or a chair or couch firmly positioned against a wall. With your arms outstretched and your back straight and in line with your legs, lean forward to grip the wall or the back of the bench, chair, or couch. Maintain tucked-in elbows while gradually lowering your weight as far as you can. Strive to lift yourself. 8 to 12 times total.

Dynamic stretches can improve flexibility, assist in warming up, and prevent injury before exercise. Without sufficient stretching or warming up, the risk of injury increases when hitting a golf ball or launching into a strenuous game of tennis. Traditional static stretching improves flexibility but is not a substitute for a warm-up. The answer is a dynamic warm-up that incorporates compound motions; in other words, moving your body while stretching.

Warm-ups that mimic your movements during the workout are the most effective. Utilizing a restricted range of motion and maintaining within your capabilities are the keys to performing dynamic warm-ups for persons with arthritis. Do a modified squat, for instance, rather than a full squat. To warm up before your next workout, try these seven dynamic stretches.

Hip Circles

Using a countertop as support, stand on one leg and slowly swing the other leg out to the side in circles. Make 20 circles, 20 in every direction. Change legs. As your flexibility improves, gradually enlarge the circles.

Arm Circles

Standing with your feet shoulder-width apart and your arms outstretched at shoulder

height with your palms down is a good posture. Make 20 arm circles, 20 in each direction. Increase the size of the circles gradually as your flexibility increases.

Arm Movements

Stand with your arms in front of you, parallel to the floor, palms down. Step forward while simultaneously swinging your arms to the right so your left arm is placed in front of your chest and your fingers are pointing in that direction. Maintain a forward-facing posture while moving just at the shoulders. As you stride again, swing your arms in the other direction. Five times on each side, repeat.

High-Steading Stand

With your right knee raised toward your chest, advance with your left leg (use a wall for balance, if needed). To raise the knee even higher, use both hands (or just one if you need the other for balance). Repeat on the other side after pausing to lower the right leg. As you advance, keep "high-stepping" five times on each leg.

Heel to Toe Walk

With your feet shoulder-width apart, stand. Take a tiny step forward, stepping onto the ball of your right foot as you plant your right heel firmly on the ground. While moving the left foot forward and taking the same heel-to-toe roll, rise as high as you can on your toes. Five times, repeat

Lunges with a Twist

Standing with your feet parallel, take a large stride forward with your right foot, fully putting it on the ground in front of you. If necessary, keep one hand on a wall for balance. Keep your torso erect and progressively bend your knee and hip. Do not let your right knee extend past your toes; keep it over your ankle. Your left knee should be a few inches above the floor as you gently bend it (or as far as flexibility allows). In this position, extend your left arm overhead (skip the overhead reach if your shoulders are unstable and slant your torso to the right. Lift your torso back up, then take a forward stride with your left foot to get back to your starting position. Five times on each side, repeat. (Note: If you struggle with balance, do not attempt this.)

Rise and Cross

Hands-on hips, feet shoulder-width apart (or lightly touching a wall in front of you for balance). Step out to the right leg as if you were stepping over something by shifting your weight to your left leg and raising your right leg until your thigh becomes parallel to the floor. Pause, then squat to the ground (or half squat). Get up by pushing through your heels, then revert to the starting posture. Five times on each side, repeat.

Remember: Know Your Limits

You can feel pain after working out if you haven't been active recently. You exercised too intensely if you were sore for longer than two hours following your workout. Consult your doctor about the types of normal pain and those that indicate a more serious condition. Ask your doctor or therapist if you should exercise during a general or local flare-up if you have rheumatoid arthritis. You can try exercising simply in your range of motion to keep your body moving while dealing with joint flare-ups, or you can exercise in water to protect your joints.

CHAPTER 4: EXERCISES TO FIGHT ARTHRITIS

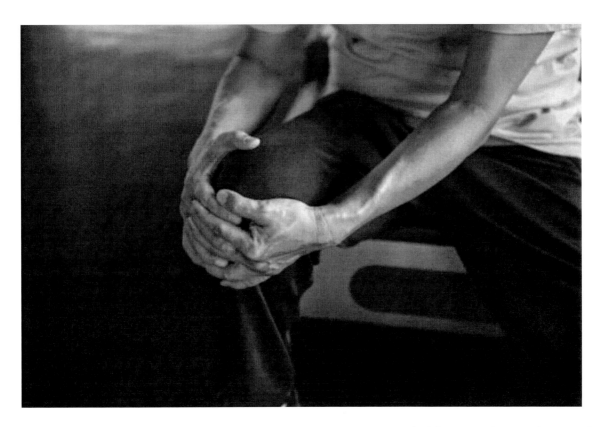

All seniors should see their doctor before starting a new arthritic exercise regimen. Before you start, your doctor might want to check your cardiovascular health, and they might have useful suggestions about the best activities for your health concerns. They might also advise you to engage with a physical therapist to discover the most effective arthritic exercises.

Spend a few minutes warming up the area of your body you'll be working on before you start your workout. Additionally, make sure you equally exercise your left and right sides. Don't forget to take the required measures, such as examining the condition of any exercise equipment or clearing enough space to avoid falls or other injuries when exercising. If you get pain while exercising, stop immediately. Seniors who struggle to exercise without pain can benefit from physical therapy.

Exercise is a good strategy to maintain fitness, keep muscles strong, and control arthritis symptoms, along with taking the right medications and giving your joints the proper amount of rest. Daily activity, such as walking or swimming, reduces discomfort, keeps joints mobile, and strengthens the muscles surrounding the joints.

According to the Arthritis Foundation, losing only 1 pound will result in a 4-pound reduction in the load on your joints. These easy arthritic exercises for seniors will help you feel better. Additionally, always remember to perform each exercise on both sides of your body to balance your training.

Hands or Wrists Exercise

Closed Fist

Maintaining finger flexibility is crucial for elderly people with arthritis in their hands. This exercise is advantageous. Simply make a fist out of your hand, moving gently if required. Make a fist out of your hand and hold it there for five seconds or as long as possible. Repeat after releasing ten times.

Wrist Flexion

Some elderly folks with arthritis find that their wrists can't bend as far or keep getting trapped. This exercise can be helpful if done frequently. Put your elbow on a table and raise your hand to the sky. Pull back your open palm gradually with your other hand. Try to push yourself as far as possible without inflicting unnecessary pain. After holding for five seconds, let go. At this moment, extend your hand, hold it for five seconds, and then release it. Then, repeat using the other hand.

Draw an "O"

If you have very severe arthritis, this final exercise could be difficult, but it can also be quite helpful. Try to form the letter "O" with your hand. Try to softly connect your thumb to your index finger while holding your fingers together and bending your thumb. With practice, you'll get better at this workout. To improve agility, try touching all your fingers to your thumb.

Exercises for the Knees

Seated Stretching

Your hips will be moved gently during this workout; as a bonus, your leg muscles will be stretched. Stretch your legs in front of you as you sit down on the ground. This stretching exercise can be done in a chair or on the bed if you cannot sit on the floor. Reaching with your hands, slowly bend forward at the hips. Don't strain yourself because you probably won't be able to reach extremely far at first. You will learn to be more adaptable over time.

Knee discomfort can be relieved by gently bending the knee. To perform this practice, no extra tools are required. Find the closest staircase instead. Step one leg on the bottom step, then the other, keeping your balance if necessary by holding on to the banister. Repetition after going back off the step.

Circular Ankles

By putting your ankle through its full range of motion, this exercise stretches your ankle joints and relaxes your muscles. Hold on to the side of a chair if you require more stability and support. Raise one foot off the ground as you stand up. Simply pointing your toe and rotating your ankle will create a circle. Make five circles, then reverse your course. Be careful when carrying out identical procedures on the opposite ankle.

Raised-Leg Position (Seated)

Straighten your back while you recline on your chair. Straighten one of your legs and lift it. Hold for a slow 10-count before lowering your leg gradually. Ten times total for each leg.

Stretching Muscles

Lay on your back with a towel rolled up beneath the ankle of one of your legs. The knee of the other leg is bent. Push the back of your knee firmly toward the bed or the floor using the muscles in your straight leg. Hold for a slow five counts. With each leg, repeat at least five times. By performing this exercise, you can keep your knee from bending all the time. Try to perform this while lying down at least once each day.

Leg Stretch

As you sit on the ground, extend your legs straight out in front of you. Slowly raise one knee to your chest while moving your foot around the floor until you feel a stretch. Hold for five seconds. Your leg should be extended as far as it can go, followed by a five-second pause. Ten times in total for one leg. If you cannot get down onto the ground, sit on a sofa and slide your foot along a board or tea tray.

Raised-Leg Position (Lying)

You can perform this while lying in bed or on the floor. Knee-bending with one leg. Lift your foot barely off the bed or floor while keeping your other leg straight. Hold for a leisurely five counts, then release. Each morning and evening, repeat the exercise five times with each leg.

Sit/Stands

Occupy a chair. Sit back down, then stand up without using your hands as a brace. Be sure to move slowly and deliberately with each step. Continue till you are unable to go on. Repeat twice more after a minute of rest. Start by standing up from a cushion on the seat if the chair is too low, then take it off after you finish.

Roll Exercises for the Quads

Stretch your legs in front of you as you sit on the floor, sofa, or bed. A towel should be placed beneath one knee. Towel pressure should resemble that of straightening your knee. Pulling your foot and toes inward will cause your calf muscles to stretch and your heel to rise off the ground. After holding for 5 seconds, take a 5-second break. After ten repetitions, switch to the other leg and repeat the exercise.

Crossed Legs

Cross your ankles while sitting on the edge of a table, seat, or bed. To make your thigh muscles tense, push your rear and front leg backward and forward against one another. As long as you can, maintain this, then unwind. Repeat this process twice, then take a minute to recover. Repeat while changing legs.

Arthritis Shoulder Exercise

Rotator Cuff and Outer Shoulder

Stand close to a counter or table. Lean forward and support yourself by resting one hand on the table. Allow the other arm to hang at your side unrestricted. Ten times, gently swing your arm forth and back. Ten times, gently swing your arm from side to side. Swing your arm ten times in a gentle circle. Continue by using the other arm. One more time, repeat the complete series. Don't lock your knees or round your back.

Crossover Arm Stretch

With your shoulders relaxed, stand straight. Pull one arm as far across your chest as is comfortable while holding it at the upper arm. Thirty seconds of stretching followed by 30 seconds of relaxation. Continue by using the other arm. Follow the same pattern three more times. Advice: Avoid pulling or applying pressure to your elbow.

Passive Internal Rotation

A yardstick, wooden dowel, or cane make good lightweight sticks. One hand should hold the stick behind your back while the other should only loosely hold the opposite end. Pull the stick horizontally to feel a pull in the front of your shoulder without experiencing any discomfort. Thirty seconds of holding is followed by 30 seconds of relaxation. On the opposite side, repeat. Follow the same pattern three more times. Advice: Avoid slouching or angling to one side while pulling the stick.

Passive External Rotation

A yardstick, wooden dowel, or cane make good lightweight sticks. Take hold of the stick with one hand and cup the other end with the other (so the stick is horizontal in front of you). Push the stick horizontally until you feel a pull at the rear of your shoulder without any discomfort while keeping the elbow of the shoulder you are extending against the side of your body. Thirty seconds of holding is followed by 30 seconds of relaxation. On the other side, repeat. Follow the same pattern three more times. Don't twist and keep your hips facing forward.

The Wall Crawl

It increases the range of motion and fortifies shoulder muscles. Place yourself in front of a wall so your fingers are just above it and about an arm's length away. Raise your fingers against the wall as comfortably as you can use the injured arm. (Refrain from shrugging toward your ear; keep your shoulder down.) Hold for 15–30 seconds, then descend by crawling. Repeat this process one or two more times, aiming higher each time.

Experts suggest pausing for a moment and concentrating on relaxing the shoulder muscle if you experience a sharp ache, or your shoulder tightens as you crawl your fingers up. Once your shoulder is at ease, you might be able to climb a little higher. If you get another cramp, you have used up your range of motion.

Wall Pushups

It bolsters the muscles of the chest, arms, and shoulders. Stand in front of the wall with your back, arms, and hands flat. Put your feet slightly farther apart than shoulder-width apart and tense your abs. Bend the elbows and open your chest toward the wall while keeping your feet flat on the floor. Slowly and carefully lower your upper body toward the wall. In the rear, your shoulder blades will slightly converge. Pause for a second. Pushing slowly until your arms are straight, push back while keeping your hands flat against the wall.

Repeat eight times, then progressively increase the number of reps. Shroyer offers the following advice: Watch out for your fingertips on the wall. Your arm, shoulder, and chest muscles are fully activated when you press firmly against the wall while maintaining them flat.

Exercises for Hip Arthritis

Here are a few workout examples for you to attempt. The exercises could be recommended to treat an ailment or for recovery. Slowly begin each exercise. If you begin to experience pain, stop doing the exercises.

Straight-Leg Raises

Lie on your side with the hip that is hurting up top. To keep your upper leg's knee straight, contract the muscles in the front of your thigh. Keep your knee pointed forward and your hip and leg straight in line with the rest of your body. Avoid leaning your hips back. About 30 centimeters off the ground, lift your top leg straight toward the ceiling. Hold for roughly 6 seconds before lowering your leg gradually. 8 to 12 times total. Even if only one hip hurts, switch legs and go through steps 1 through 5 again.

Internal Straight-Leg Lifts

Lie on your side with the hip that is hurting flat on the ground. You can either bend and place that foot in front of your other knee or support your other leg on a chair. Avoid leaning your hips back. To straighten the knee on your bottom leg, contract the muscles in front of your thigh. Lift your lower leg toward the ceiling by about 15 centimeters while keeping your kneecap pointed front and your leg straight. Hold for roughly 6 seconds, then gradually descend. 8 to 12 times total. Even if only one hip hurts, switch legs and go through steps 1 through 5 again.

Swag Hike

Hold onto the wall or banister while standing sideways on the bottom step of a staircase. Lift your good leg off the step and let it hang down while keeping both knees straight. Then, raise your healthy hip to, or just above, the level of your injured hip. 8 to 12 times total. Even if only one hip hurts, switch legs and go through steps 1 through 3 again.

Bridging

Kneel on your back with both of them bent. Your knees have to be bent 90 degrees. Plant your feet firmly on the ground, tighten your buttocks, and lift your hips off the floor when your shoulders, hips, and knees are straight.

Hamstring Flex (Lying Down)

Straighten your legs as you lay flat on your back. Put a small towel roll under your lower back if you experience back pain. Holding the back of the injured leg, raise it straight up and toward your body until the back of your thigh stretches. For at least 30 seconds, maintain the stretch. Do this exercise 2 to 4 times. Even if only one hip hurts, switch legs and go through steps 1 through 4 again.

Quadriceps Stretch while Standing

Hold on to a chair, counter, or wall if your balance is shaky. To perform this exercise, you can lie on your side or stomach. Stretching a leg involves bending the knee and reaching back with the same-side hand to grab the front of the foot or ankle. For example, use your right hand to extend your right leg. Pull your foot toward your buttock while keeping your knees close together until you feel a light stretch over the front of your hip and down the front of your thigh. Instead of pointing out to the side, your knee should be squarely toward the ground. For at least 15-30 seconds, maintain the stretch. Do this exercise 2 to 4 times. Even if only one hip hurts, switch legs and go through steps 1 through 5 again.

Hip Rotator Stretching

Place your feet flat on the floor as you lay on your back with both knees bent. Put the injured leg's ankle on the thigh opposite to the knee. Until you feel a light stretch around your hip, use your hand to gently press your knee away from your body. For 15 to 30 seconds, maintain the stretch. Do this exercise 2 to 4 times. Repetition of steps 1 through 5 with the addition of a gentle hand-pull of the opposing knee toward the opposite shoulder.

Knee-to-Chest

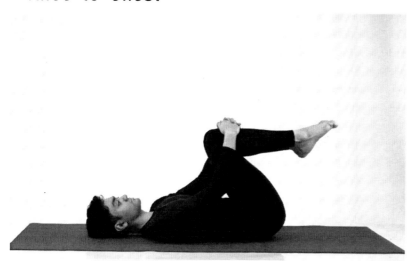

Keep your feet flat on the floor as you lay on your back with your knees bent. Keep the other foot flat while you lift the injured leg to your chest (or keep the other leg straight, whichever feels better on your lower back). Hold your lower back firmly against the floor. Hold for between 15 and 30 seconds, minimum. Remain calm and bring your knee back to its original position. Do this exercise 2 to 4 times. Even if only one hip hurts, switch legs and go through steps 1 through 5 again. Set the other leg flat on the floor and draw your knee to your chest for greater stretch.

Clamshell

Lie on your side with the hip that is hurting up top. Keep your knees bent, and your feet and legs close together. Your top knee should be raised while maintaining a close foot spacing.

Avoid rolling your hips back. Your legs should be apart like clams. Take a 6-second hold. Bring your knee back down gradually. Take a 10-second break. 8 to 12 times total.

CHAPTER 5: ROUTINE EXERCISES

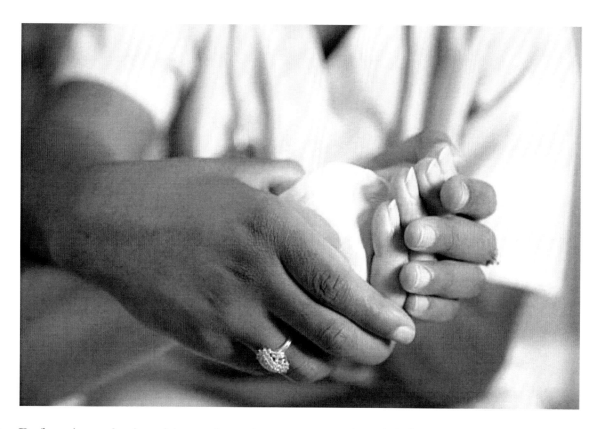

Note: Before introducing this workout into your routine, it is best to consult your doctor first and get his approval.

Full Body Workout

This workout covers all the different parts of the body, so if you have arthritis pain in any particular area of the body, say just the knees, this workout routine will still help you to reduce the pain and fight the stiffness.

Warm-Up

1. **Sit Stand:** 2 minutes
2. **Leg Figure Eights:** 60 seconds
3. **Hip Circles:** 60 seconds
4. **Arm Circles:** 60 seconds
5. **Heel to Toe Walk:** 2 minutes

Workout

1. **Closed Fist:** 10 Reps
2. **Wrist Flexion:** 2 sets of 10 Reps
3. **Seated Stretching:** 10 Reps
4. **Raised-Leg Position (Seated):** 10 Reps each leg
5. **The Wall Crawl:** 10 Reps
6. **Wall Pushups:** 10 Reps
7. **Bridging:** 20 Reps
8. **Clamshell:** 10 Reps
9. **Rotator Cuff and Outer Shoulder:** 10 reps

Cool Down

1. **Lunges With a Twist:** 60 seconds
2. **Rise And Cross:** 60 seconds

BOOK 6:
SCIATICA EXERCISES
FOR SENIORS

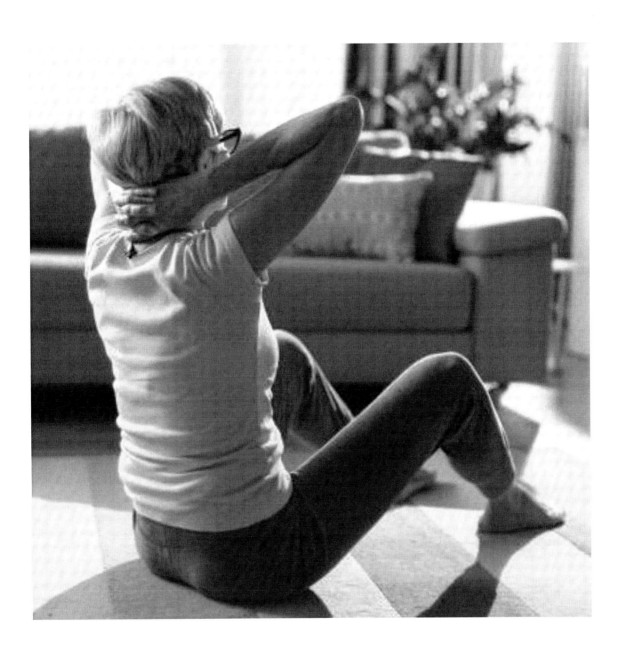

CHAPTER 1: UNDERSTANDING SCIATICA

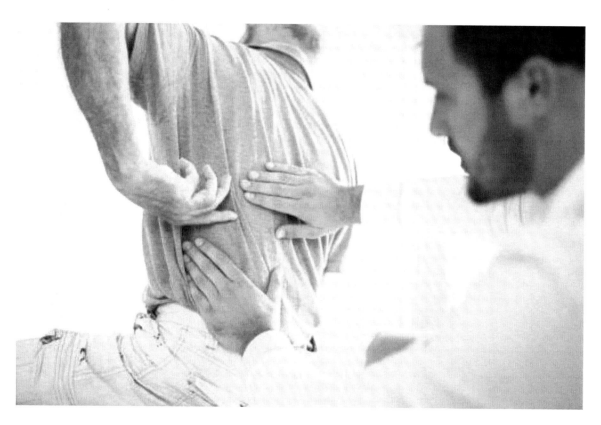

Back pain can take many different forms. It may start to hurt immediately or develop slowly and erratically over several months. It could be sudden, brief (acute), or persistent (chronic). Some back pain can be treated with over-the-counter medications, but others can only be treated with strong medications or surgery. Sometimes it's challenging to pinpoint the cause of your back discomfort, while other times, it's simple. One of those that is quite easy to recognize is sciatica. You might not even need to call a doctor because home cures might be effective quickly.

Your lumbar (lower) spine's herniated disc is the typical source of sciatica. Round, flat, flexible discs of connective tissue separate and protect the vertebrae, the bones that make up your spine. A disk's soft center may protrude from the hard outer ring as it becomes worn down, whether from years of use or an injury. The nerves nearby may experience pressure if a disc herniates.

The longest nerve in your body is the sciatic nerve. It originates in your lower back and divides to travel down both sides of your hips, buttocks, legs, and feet. The sciatic nerve in the lower back may also experience pressure from bone spurs and spinal stenosis (narrowing). When it occurs, there may be several issues that extend down the nerve. Pain that extends from your lower back into the back or side of your legs is the most recognizable sign of sciatica. It may be a dull discomfort or a strong, excruciating agony. Your leg or foot may also experience numbness, tingling, and weakness.

Risk Factors

- **Age.** The majority of sciatica sufferers are between the ages of 30 and 50.
- **Weight.** Being overweight or pregnant increases the pressure on your spine, which increases your risk of developing a herniated disc.
- **Diabetes:** Nerve injury can result from diabetes.
- **Work.** A lot of hard lifting or extended periods of sitting might harm discs.

Treatment

Most sciatica sufferers recover without surgery in a few weeks. Ibuprofen (Advil) and naproxen sodium (Aleve), available over the counter, can also aid pain management, but they should only be used temporarily.

Additionally, your doctor could advise using cold packs for your lower back for a few days before transitioning to hot packs for additional few days. There are numerous effective stretches to alleviate sciatica and lower back pain.

When you have sciatica, your initial inclination might be to rest and take it easy, but maintaining movement is more crucial. The nerve in that location will remain inflamed if you remain stationary. The irritation will be lessened by continuing to move.

Your doctor will likely recommend stronger medication, such as anti-inflammatories or muscle relaxants if home cures don't work. You could also try chiropractic treatment, physical therapy, acupuncture, or steroid injections. It might be time for surgery if your pain persists for more than three months. If your sciatica produces excruciating pain, weakness, numbness, or loss of bladder or bowel control, see your doctor right once.

Non-Medicinal Treatments of Sciatica

The greater risk of complications is considered while developing treatment protocols for low back pain in older persons. The main recommendations focus on pain control and gradual, regulated, and regular exercise. A healthy amount of activity also aids in avoiding unanticipated consequences like pressure sores from prolonged bed rest or psychological distress brought on by insufficient daily activity and a decline in endorphin production. Simply stretching is far preferable to bed rest on days when pain is acute, and exercise seems impossible.

Ice Therapy

An increase in inflammation usually accompanies most episodes of severe low back pain. Inflammation with cold therapy, such as a disposable ice pack or frozen veggie bag, will decrease. To reduce inflammation after physical activity or exercise, it is often advised to immediately administer ice therapy (cryotherapy) for 20 minutes at a time, as needed, every 2 hours. Since the skin may be in danger of further harm, ice therapy may not be advised for elderly people with diabetes or other nerve problems.

Heat Therapy

Osteoarthritis-related stiffness or muscle spasms are usually linked to low back discomfort. Applying heat to the lower back will relax the muscles and expand the range of motion, effectively treating both spasms and stiffness. Using heat packs for around 20 minutes is advised before strenuous exercise or physical activity. People with specific skin diseases, such as dermatitis, heart issues, or diabetes, may not be advised to use heat therapy.

Exercise: Controlled and Progressive

Almost all treatment plans for lower back pain incorporate frequent, controlled, and progressive exercise as part of their physical therapy regimen. Back pain in older people is rarely treated; instead, it is usually lessened or made more manageable so that everyday activities can be performed more easily and with more function.

One to two hours of cardiovascular exercise, such as brisk walking, and two days of strength training per week are generally advised for older persons.

Committing to regular exercise is crucial because these workout routines work best when followed for at least six weeks. Compared to youth, recuperation times are typically lengthier as people get older. For older persons, the following are practical, simple, and effective activities:

Water Exercise

Warm swimming pool exercises are just as beneficial as other supervised exercises at home, during physical treatment, or in a gym. For elderly folks, the water environment's buoyancy is a safer substitute. Exercises in the water often result in less severe initial soreness and stiffness. Additionally, aquatic treatment lessens melancholy and anxiety while enhancing balance, flexibility, and function.

Exercises for Lumbar Stabilization

Dynamic stability exercises help older persons build stronger muscles and improve their capacity to prevent falls and regain their balance after a fall. This type of exercise has a 30% reduction in pain and impairment. Five exercises to strengthen the core. Low back pain is thought to be reduced by exercises that stabilize and strengthen the trunk muscles, especially as part of an extensive physical treatment regimen. Increasing general stability, posture, and steadiness while walking can be achieved by strengthening the core muscles.

Certain workouts may be more or less suitable depending on the underlying disease. The exercises listed below might not be appropriate for all patients.

- Osteoporosis sufferers should avoid yoga poses that require full forward- or backward-bends or hip rotation.

- For someone with degenerative spondylolisthesis or lumbar spinal stenosis, backward-bending exercises may be unpleasant.

- A person with a disc issue in their lower back may not be advised to perform exercises that require bending forward at the waist.

- Some flexibility-focused workouts can put too much stress on the spine and exacerbate back pain.

It is recommended to begin any new stretching or exercise routine under the direction of a licensed healthcare provider. Easy-to-do exercises and gentle and low-intensity activities are more likely to be maintained over time. Starting a new fitness program for older persons who have little to no physical activity will probably need assistance from a certified specialist, such as a physical trainer, physical therapist, or physiatrist.

Healthy Eating for Sciatica

Magnesium helps your body release muscle contractions; thus, it is typically advised for persons with sciatica to eat meals high in this mineral. Approximately 99 percent of the total magnesium in your body is stored in your bones, muscles, and soft tissues, with only about 1 percent of it being concentrated in the blood.

Foods rich in magnesium include Swiss chard, spinach, dark chocolate, dried pumpkin seeds, black beans, avocado, dried figs, yogurt, bananas, dairy, apricots, fish, and brown rice. Consuming more of these foods can help you manage and relieve sciatic pain. People with sciatica also eat omega-3-, vitamin b-, and antioxidant-rich foods, all of which help reduce the inflammation associated with this condition.

You must consume extra omega-3 essential fatty acids since they naturally lower inflammation. Salmon, fish, sardines, and cold-water fish are all edible, the speaker asserts. You should cut out any additional animal protein from your diet. Eat more veggies and foods high in B vitamins. Consume many foods high in fiber, such as whole grains, legumes, and cereals. These offer a lot of phytonutrients and antioxidants. As you make dietary adjustments, limit your calorie intake because weight gain might exacerbate this illness.

Exercise and Activity Can Help Manage Pain

While it may seem sensible to rest your body when you have sciatica to avoid any kind of flare-up, prolonged inactivity might exacerbate the condition. To help you keep active while managing sciatica, discuss building a personalized activity plan with your doctor or other healthcare professional. Remember to stick to the plan because the inappropriate activity will probably worsen your sciatica pain and last longer.

From a fitness perspective, the ideal workouts for reducing sciatica pain and bolstering the muscles that support your spine entail exercising your core. Here are a few distinct exercises that are great for those who are currently experiencing sciatica pain:

- **Walking.** Walking for 30 minutes daily is the best exercise for the lower back and offers the same benefits as one aerobic exercise session.
- **Swimming.** Swimming is a low-impact workout that increases heart rate, aids calorie burning, and is mild on the spine. Swimming laps across the pool, water strolling, or aqua aerobics are all options.
- **Pilates.** Pilates, which focuses on developing and enhancing mental sharpness and core strength, supports the maintenance of a well-aligned spine. Pilates involves your body in movement that is deliberate and controlled. Similar to swimming, it has low impact and aids in body shaping and toning.
- **Yoga.** Yoga poses that are gentle on the back include the cat-cow sequence, child's pose, and upward-facing dog. Numerous fundamental postures assist you in freeing up

your back and stretching any muscles that may have gotten stiff and tight from sitting while also providing rapid pain relief.

- **Stretching.** Stretching every day before getting out of bed might ease sciatica pain by preparing the muscles

Exercises to Stay Away From

Pay attention to your body's signals and avoid any painful activities. Certain workouts might worsen sciatica symptoms, especially if they put pressure or strain on your legs, core, or back. Although it's crucial to improve your strength and flexibility in these areas, you must do so gradually and sensibly.

Avoid high-impact activities because they can exacerbate injuries and symptoms. If you're in a lot of pain, stop doing what you're doing. Try stretching gently or exercising whenever possible to avoid worsening your symptoms.

CHAPTER 2: WARM-UP AND COOL-DOWN EXERCISES

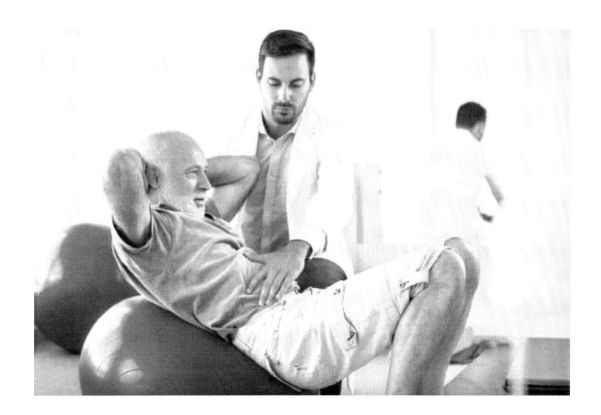

Forward Bend

Take a deep breath and raise your arms overhead while lifting and lengthening your head's crown and fingers. On an exhalation, progressively descend the torso toward the legs while hunching at the hips. Reach your hands down to your ankles, feet, or toes. Pull the head and body closer to the legs using your arms to deepen the stretch. Extend your heels and softly pull your toes toward you. For 3 to 8 breaths, hold your breath. Release: Return to Staff stance while slowly rolling up the spine. As you elevate your torso back into Staff pose, exhale while bringing your arms back over your head.

Two-Hurdler Stretch

Place one leg straight in front of you as you sit on the floor. Bend the knee of your remaining leg, so your foot is behind your torso, and your thigh points out to the side. Your physique will resemble that of a hurdler. Hold this posture while reaching your hands toward the toes of the extended leg in front of your body while leaning your chest forward. Hold the position for 30 seconds before switching to the other leg.

Circular Leg Raises

One technique to make the leg raise simpler is to bend your knees while performing it; however, lifting one limb at a time is also a less strenuous option. Keep one leg on the ground to keep your body stable while raising the other leg and concentrating on your form.

Simple Stretch in Chair

First, sit on a chair with your hurting leg crossed over the knee of the opposite leg. Bend your chest forward while keeping your back and spine straight. Bend a little further forward if no pain is felt. For around 30 seconds, maintain this posture. Stretch your second leg out in the same manner.

Buttock Stretch

Bring your knees to your chest while lying on your back. Cross your left thigh across the right leg. Take both hands and grasp the back of your left leg. Draw your left leg close to your heart. Continue with the other leg.

Front Thigh

For this stretch of the front thigh muscles, bring your heel towards your buttocks.

Grasp your heel with your hands and push your pelvis slightly forward until you feel a pleasant pull in the thigh.

Forward Fold

The forward fold is a great full-body exercise to begin your cool-down stretching regimen. To melt your torso down until your hands are on—or reaching toward—the floor, stand with your feet hip-width apart and reach up to the ceiling. Be sure to squat with your knees bent as far as necessary and allow your head to hang loosely for a moment. It also feels great to shake your head in a "yes" and "no" manner.

Reclined Twist

The reclined twist is a miracle stretch for the spine. It feels great, releases tons of tension, and is an incredible tool for winding down from a killer workout. Lay flat on your back with both legs straight out. Bring one knee to your chest, grab it with your hands, and gently guide it to the opposite side of your body until it reaches (or gets close to) the floor. Once your leg is across your torso, you can release your hands and put your arms straight to the sides. For a little extra stretch, turn your head in the opposite direction of your bent, crossed knee. Repeat on the other side and enjoy.

Side Reach

This simple side stretch gets to all the intercostal muscles supporting your torso. Stand with your feet wider than shoulder-width apart. Put one hand on your hip and the other up and over your head toward the opposite corner of the ceiling. You can also do this with both hands clasped and your index fingers pointing up. Breathe into that side body and repeat.

CHAPTER 3: EXERCISES TO FIGHT SCIATICA

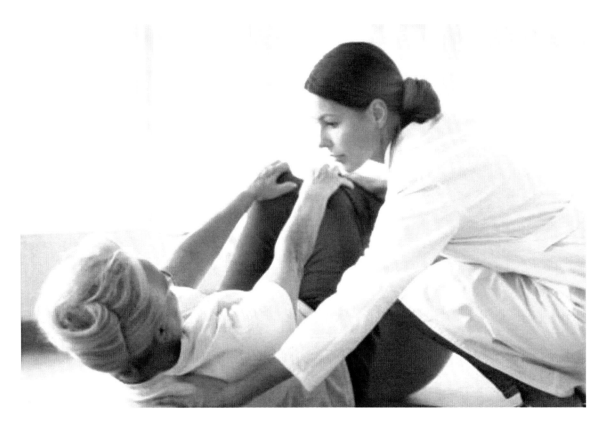

A list of best exercises against sciatica and general exercises that help with sciatica back pain.

Squats with Weights

Weighted squats increase compression on your intervertebral discs, nerves, and lower back. They might also exert pressure on your legs, causing harm and agony. Try them without the weights, keeping your back neutral and your core engaged. If you experience any back discomfort or tightness, stop.

Sit and Stretch Your Glutes

For the seated glute stretch, you must sit cross-legged. As you sit on the ground, extend your legs straight out in front of you. Bend your right leg and keep your right ankle on your left knee. Leaning forward, let your upper body slope toward your thigh. Hold for 15 to 30 seconds. This stretches the glutes and lower back. Repeat on the other side.

Seated Spinal Flexion

Turn to your side to prevent the sciatic nerve from being squeezed while completing the sitting spinal stretch. Compression of the spine's vertebrae results in sciatica pain. You can reduce the pressure on the sciatic nerve by stretching the spine. Sit down on the mat on the floor with your legs extended in front of you and your feet flexed upward. While bending your right knee, place your right foot outside your left knee. Put your left elbow outside your right knee and slowly move your body to the right. A side switch comes after holding for 30 seconds each three times.

Basic Seated Stretch

Keep your back straight as you extend each leg in the basic seated stretch. Sit on a chair and cross the knee of your hurting leg over the knee of the other leg to begin this stretch. After that, do the following: While leaning forward with your chest, try to keep your spine straight. If it doesn't hurt, try bending over a little bit more. When you feel any pain, stop. Thirty seconds in this position, then switch to the other leg and repeat the exercise with that leg.

Stretch Figure 4

The figure-4 stance can be used to stretch the piriformis muscle. The figure-4 stretch might help you open your hips. While flat on your back, bend both your knees. Cross your right foot across your left thigh as you bring your legs up toward your torso. After briefly maintaining the position, switch to the other side. During this stage, you must be careful not to strain. Allow gravity to naturally bring your legs closer to your body so you may extend further.

Knee to the Other Shoulder

You lay flat and extend your leg to the opposite shoulder. This simple stretch helps reduce sciatica pain by loosening your gluteal and piriformis muscles, which can swell and press against the sciatic nerve. Lying calmly on your back with your legs outstretched and your feet flexed upward. When you bend your right leg, your hands should be about the knee. Cross your right leg over to your left shoulder while gently pulling. Hold it for another 30 seconds. Just pull your knee as far as it can go comfortably, remember. Your muscle should just feel a soothing stretch rather than any discomfort. Pushing your knee will cause your leg to revert to its original position. Change legs after three repetitions.

The Pigeon Pose in Front

Squat on the ground with your knees bent to begin this version of the pigeon stance. Kneel on the ground while on all fours. Pick up your right leg and move it on the ground in front of your torso. Your lower leg should be parallel to your torso and flat on the ground. Your right knee should stay to the right, and your left knee should be behind your right foot. The left leg should be extended behind you, with the toes pointed back and the top of the foot on the floor.

Gradually shift your body weight so that your legs bear most of your weight rather than your arms. Put your hands on either side of your legs as you sit up straight. Breathe in deeply. Lean your upper body over your front leg as you exhale. With your support, your weight. Repeat on the other side.

Hamstring Stretch while Standing

To complete the standing hamstring stretch, start by standing up and placing your right foot on something higher, like a chair. This stretch may help with hamstring tightness and pain brought on by sciatica. Place your right foot at hip height or lower on an elevated surface. This could be a stair step, an ottoman, or a chair. Flex your foot to extend your leg and toes. If your knee tends to hyperextend, keep it slightly bent. Arc your body forward slightly in the direction of your foot. The stretch deepens as you move on. Avoid pushing yourself past your pain threshold. Release your elevated leg's hip downward rather than raise it. If you need help bringing your hip down, wrap a yoga strap or long exercise band around your right thigh and under your left foot. Hold for at least 30 seconds, then switch to the other side.

Piriformis Stretch while Standing

You can provide more stability to the standing piriformis stretch by resting your hands on your hips. This is another standing stretch that relieves sciatica pain. You can do this independently; if not, you can lean on a wall with your feet about 24 inches away. Cross the knee of the painful leg across the other while you're standing. Try to form the number 4 while bending your standing leg and bringing your hips down to the ground at a 45-degree angle. Bend at the waist while maintaining a straight back, then swing your arms. For 30 to 60 seconds, maintain the position. Continue while switching legs.

Hamstring Stretch with Scissors

By squatting while completing the scissor hamstring stretch, you can reduce the pressure the hamstring muscles place on the sciatic nerve. The ischial tuberosity, often referred to as the sit or sitz bones starts at the ischium, one of the pelvic girdle's three main structural elements, along with the ilium and the pubis. The ischial tuberosity and the hamstring muscles are connected by the sacrotuberous ligament (STL). When hamstring muscles are tight, they can mirror sciatica symptoms. This stretch can help those hamstring muscles unwind, releasing some strain on the sciatic nerve. Utilizing this activity every day could be advantageous.

Pelvic Tilt

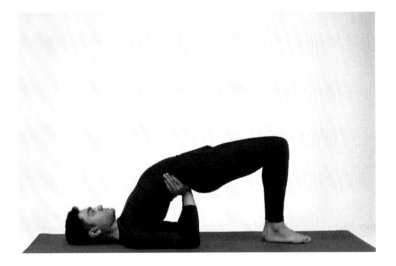

This stretch can be performed on a hard mattress if that is more convenient for you; however, a yoga mat is recommended. Initially, lie on your back. Bend your knees and place your feet flat on the ground with your toes pointed forward. Pull your belly button in, flatten your back on the floor, and lift your pelvis toward the ceiling. Relax in this position after 20 seconds. If you can, repeat this stretch ten times. Be cautious about focusing on your core muscles rather than using your legs to push when tilting your pelvis.

The bridge is a similar exercise to the pelvic tilt. Start by lying down on your back with your knees bent and your feet flat on the ground. As you slowly push your buttocks up by squeezing your heels, lift your pelvis toward the ceiling. Once your thighs and torso are lined up, hold this stretch for 8 to 10 seconds (less if you're just starting), and then slowly return to the starting position.

Supine Leg Lift

The prone leg raise is a highly effective stabilizing exercise for people with sciatica pain brought on by degenerative disc degeneration. Lie prone and flat on your stomach on a yoga mat or a mattress surface. Your face should be resting on your outstretched arms in front of you. Your lower abdominal muscles ought to be tight. Raise a leg behind you with a slight bend in the knee without hunching your neck or back. Your leg should be low and not stick out much from the ground. Hold for around 5 seconds before easing back to the starting position. As your strength grows, try to complete two sets of 10-leg raises.

Remember: Exercise with Care

The stretches and exercises mentioned above may not provide pain alleviation for everyone. However, they are worth attempting and exploring with your doctor or physical therapist. Don't think you can get into these postures based on what you see on TV. Most of the workout demonstrators have years of practice and are exceptionally flexible. If you have any pain, stop doing everything. There is no one-size-fits-all exercise program for people with sciatic nerve irritation.

Making slight adjustments to the positions, such as pulling your knees in more or less, is advised, and you should do so to feel how it feels. If a person feels better, that is the treatment a person wants to follow. Anyone who has experienced slight sciatic nerve soreness for longer than a month should see a doctor or physiotherapist. An at-home workout program designed specifically for discomfort may provide you with relief.

CHAPTER 4: ROUTINE EXERCISES

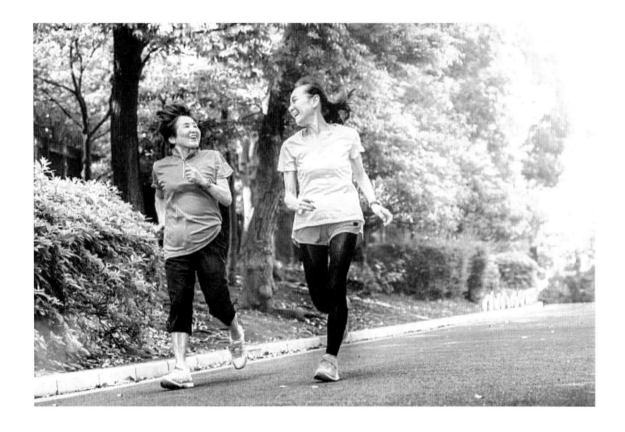

Sciatica Reliever

Warm and cold compresses before and after this exercise routine can help with the pain. Be careful while sitting in any position; evenly divide the weight on your back to avoid straining any muscle.

Warm-Up

1. **Forward bend:** 60 seconds
2. **Two-Hurdler Stretch:** 60 seconds
3. **Circular Leg Raises**: 30 seconds

Workout

1. **Hamstring Stretch while Standing**: 10 Reps
2. **Sit and Stretch your Glutes:** 10 Reps
3. **Seated Spinal Flexion**: 10 Reps
4. **Basic Seated Stretch:** 10 Reps
5. **Pelvic Tilt:** 10 Reps

Cool Down

1. **Simple Stretch in Chair:** 60 seconds
2. **Front Thigh:** 60 seconds
3. **Forward Fold:** 60 seconds

Note: Couple these exercises with doctor-suggested medicines and non-medicinal therapies to relieve the pain.

Spinal Strengthening

Don't sit too long during the exercises or throughout the day. Sitting in one position for longer than 30 minutes can increase the pain.

Warm-Up

Forward Bend: 60 seconds

Buttock Stretch: 60 seconds

Side Reach: 60 seconds

Workout

1. **Pelvic Tilt:** 15 Reps
2. **Knee to the Other Shoulder:** 10 Reps on each side
3. **The Pigeon Pose in Front:** 60 seconds
4. **Seated Spinal Flexion:** 20 Reps
5. **Supine Leg lift:** 10 Reps on each side

Cool Down

1. **Circular Leg Raises:** 60 seconds
2. **Reclined Twist:** 60 seconds

Note: Employ the back stretches from book two if you want to keep your spine more flexible and better suited for these exercises.

BOOK 7:
CHAIR YOGA FOR SENIORS

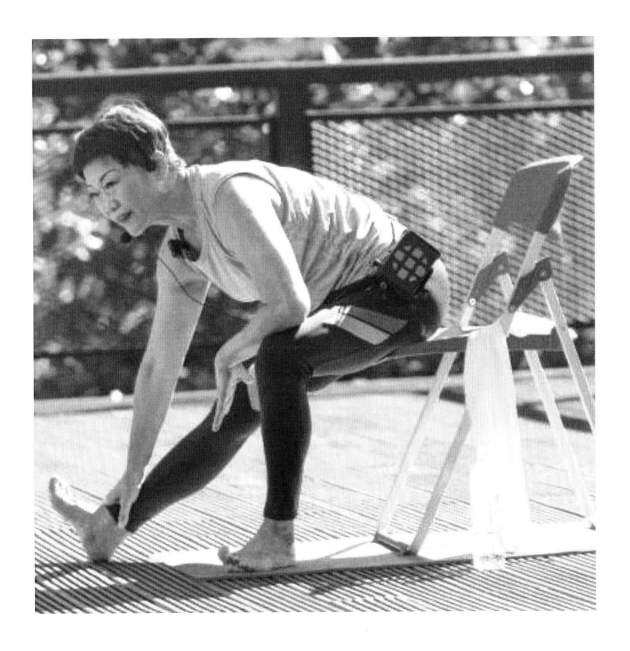

CHAPTER 1: CHAIR YOGA

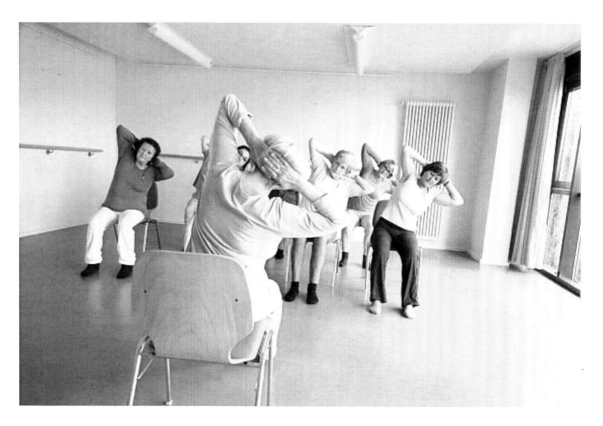

The advantages of yoga range from increased flexibility to pain alleviation. Therefore, it should be no surprise that over 90% of Americans practice yoga for health and wellness. However, traditional yoga may be challenging for some people with limited mobility and chronic illnesses like arthritis or heart disease. Fortunately, chair yoga might be a useful substitute. It includes seated yoga poses that open up the practice. Read on to learn more about chair yoga, including the essential positions.

How is Chair Yoga Performed?

This gentle practice adapts common yoga positions so you can perform them while seated in a chair. Alternatively, you can maintain your balance while practicing standing poses by using a chair. Most positions, including twists, backbends, and forward folds, can be modified for chair yoga. Therefore, you can enroll in a chair yoga class or a regular yoga class with adjustments for sitting poses that are appropriate for your fitness level.

What Advantages Does Chair Yoga Offer?

Modified chair poses also work the same muscles as regular yoga postures. Therefore, inclusive practice offers comparable health advantages. By doing chair yoga, one can:

Increase Your Flexibility and Balance

For health and well-being, maintaining balance and flexibility is essential. Doing so can lower your risk of injury and maintain your independence as you age. This is crucial because 3 million older persons visit the emergency room each year after suffering injuries from falls.

Increase Strength and Muscle Tone

People of all ages may become stronger with traditional yoga. Chair yoga could aid in developing and maintaining muscle strength in older persons. Additionally, researchers discovered that exercising in a chair enhances upper- and lower-body functionality. Because muscle mass decreases with aging, this is significant. And in older persons, that deterioration may be followed by a loss of strength and function.

Boost Your Disposition and Mental Health

Yoga practice may positively affect mental health, such as reduced anxiety and improved mood. There is evidence that these advantages hold for numerous types of yoga, including chair yoga.

Assist in Managing Chronic Illnesses

People with chronic health issues like Type 2 diabetes may benefit from seated yoga. For instance, a pilot study examined the impact of a 10-minute chair yoga session on diabetics. In addition to receiving standard care, participants were urged to follow the routine regularly.

They displayed improvements in their blood pressure, heart rate, and blood sugar in a 3-month follow-up.

Minimize Persistent Discomfort

Roughly 20% of adults experience chronic pain that can hinder their daily lives. And ongoing research shows that yoga may be an effective alternative for chronic pain management. Practicing chair yoga may help older adults reduce pain and fatigue from osteoarthritis.

Anyone Can Do Chair Yoga

Chair yoga is accessible to all. However, the modified technique might be ideal for some groups, such as:

- **People 65 Years of Age and Older:** Chair yoga is a secure, low-impact activity that can support healthy aging. Older folks may find it particularly alluring due to its adaptability and advantages, including decreased fall risk and increased functional mobility.

- **People with Chronic Health Issues:** Research suggests that seated yoga practices can help people manage chronic disorders like arthritis, diabetes, and dementia (and the discomfort that goes along with them).

- **People with Limited Mobility:** Traditional yoga's benefits are available to those with mobility issues through seated positions. For instance, chair yoga has been proven beneficial for persons healing from spinal cord injuries and multiple sclerosis.

- **People with Office Jobs:** Long periods spent at a desk can wear you out, raise your blood pressure, and hurt your lower back, neck, and Shoulders. Workplace yoga sessions could reduce back pain and improve mental health. An office chair yoga session of just 15 minutes can reduce physical and mental stress. Even so, it's best to see your doctor before beginning chair yoga, particularly if you have any health issues or diseases.

How Usually Should Chair Yoga Be Practiced?

The frequency of chair yoga sessions is not specified in any formal guidelines. However, 65 and older can perform strengthening exercises twice a week and balance exercises thrice. Therefore, beginning with two to three weekly chair yoga sessions may be a good idea. But keep in mind that any activity is preferable to none. Studies suggest that older persons may benefit from even occasional yoga sessions.

Advantages of Yoga and Breathing Deeply

Most of us are too mentally and physically rigid and fixed from our hectic lifestyles for deep breathing to have beneficial effects. Asana is useful in this situation. The asanas' physical movement helps us become less rigid and more flexible, which promotes the free flow of energy throughout the body. To assist the flow of energy through the body, each asana's physical movements are designed to be performed.

Yoga can be done in as many different positions as desired. However, the practice won't benefit the body if deep breathing isn't happening. The movement of energy and the aid in physical relaxation is brought about by breathing. A body that is already rigid will only hurt itself when it tries to assume other positions. But when we breathe deeply, we can feel more emotion and become more aware of how our bodies feel. Deep breathing during yoga can prevent damage.

Additionally, deep breathing might help us discover our inner selves. Breathing regularly induces a flow that prompts a shift in the body and mind, purifying and sanitizing them so that our actual essence emerges. Increased circulation, hormonal harmony, organ regeneration, and nervous system tranquilization all occur.

Anyone who wants a decent physical workout might only perform the positions. But yoga is meant to be so much more. We can access our transforming potential by breathing deeply.

It introduces us to yoga's capacity to refresh and shape our bodies and brains. Finally, deep breathing aids in our journey toward unification.

A strong chair without armrests or wheels, like a dining room chair, is what we advise. Your thighs must be parallel to the floor for perfect alignment to feel secure, grounded, and in control of your activity. Place a folded blanket under your seat or at your feet if your knees are pointing up or down while seated in a chair.

How Safe is Chair Yoga?

Comparing Chair Yoga to other yoga forms, it is generally believed that it has a lesser risk and lower impact. Chair yoga might be a good alternative for you if you're expecting a baby or recovering from an accident. Nevertheless, we advise you to get the go-ahead for exercise from a medical professional or physical therapist.

CHAPTER 2: CHAIR YOGA STARTING EXERCISES

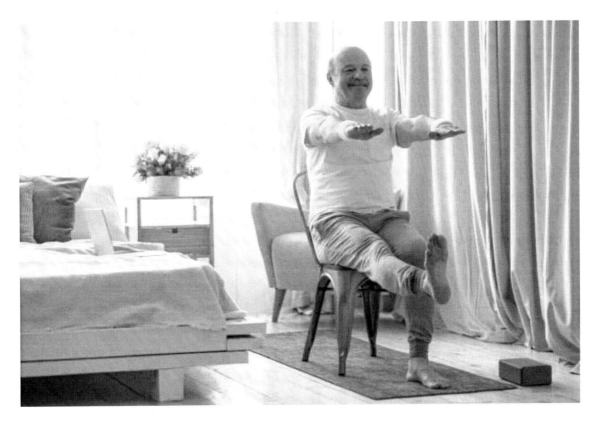

It's a great idea to speak with your doctor before starting any new workout program to receive a medical clearance and discuss any potential issues or adjustments that may be required, especially if you are over 40 or have any pre-existing medical ailments. Once you've been given the all-clear to begin chair yoga, you can practice at home or in a chair yoga class.

Aside from comfortable clothing, slip-resistant shoes or socks to prevent falls, a water bottle to stay hydrated, and a towel in case you sweat or want more padding, all you need to bring to a chair yoga class is yourself. You'll need the necessary tools to practice chair yoga at home. The right chair will minimize your chance of injury and help you get the most out of your activity. Use a sturdy, armless chair that won't rock, wobble, or wheel. Ensure your training area is level and flat so the chair is flush with the floor. The chair should be placed where there is enough room to move around it and extend your limbs in all directions without running into anything.

Breathe

Begin with a blank canvas: Place your hands on your waist and lean back in your chair. Breathe in through your nose, allowing your sides and belly to expand, gently letting it out. Repeat ten times.

Sit in a Chair

Start by sitting in your chair with your knees aligned with your hips and your feet hip-width apart. Put your hands on your knees and begin to breathe deeply. Your abdominal muscles will become more active as a result.

Thoracic Rotations in Position One

To turn your upper body to the side, place your hands on each side of your head. Hold for a short while before turning to face the opposite side.

Ragdoll

Spread your legs as wide as you can by separating your feet. Slowly bend down your spine when your head hangs between your legs. Bring your arms into position while you do this. After that, slowly swing from one side to the other while feeling your lower back extend. When finished, return to the center, roll up, and let your arms hang loose.

Side Flexes

Lean to one side while raising your other arm above your head and sliding your hand down the inside of your calf. Return to the center after feeling the stretch.

Circular Arms

Bring your feet back together, lift one of them, place your outstretched knee on the thigh of the other, and feel the stretch. If you want to intensify the stretch, stoop forward.

Tree Posture

Open and close your leg after drawing your foot up the inside of your calf. Rotate your leg from the hip joint to avoid twisting your entire body. If you require support, use the chair.

Squats

Standing up straight and put your fingertips mere inches from your chair. When squatting, push back up through your glutes while putting weight on your heels.

Backstretch

Stretch your back by bending forward and using the back of your chair as support. To achieve a deeper stretch, shift your weight from your left to your right arm while you stretch. Drop to the ground and roll up through your spine slowly.

Salutations of the Sun

Taking a deep breath, raise your arms aloft while sitting tall. Float your arms back down to your sides as you exhale. Five times. Doing so can stretch your spine and reduce neck and shoulder stress.

Cat/Cow

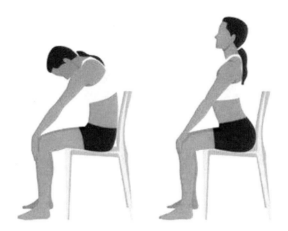

Because it lengthens and extends the spine, this chair yoga pose is excellent for the elderly, people with low back discomfort or stiffness, or people with bad postures. Sit tall, with your core engaged, shoulders back, and chest raised, with your legs on the edge of the seat. Your feet should be placed on the floor with your toes pointing forward, and your knees should be squarely over your ankles. Your hands should be placed on top of parallel, evenly separated thighs.

Inhale and assume the cow position by rolling your shoulders back and down and arching your spine. As you exhale, assume the cat position by bending your spine, shifting your shoulders forward, and lowering your chin toward your chest. Switch between the two positions for ten breaths

CHAPTER 3: CHAIR YOGA EXERCISES

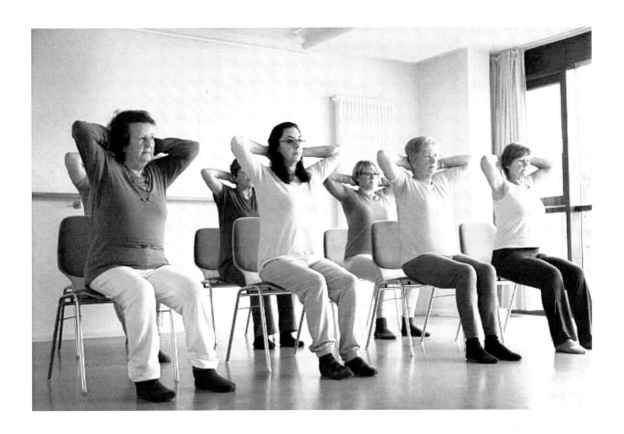

Twisted Sun Salutations

As you exhale, carry out the preceding exercise with a twist. On each side, repeat the procedure five times, holding the final twist for five seconds.

Altar Side Leans High

Raise your arms over your head and entwine your fingers in front of you for a powerful spine and shoulder stretch. Next, straighten your arms above your head while turning your palms upward. For three breaths, lean to the right, then for three to the left.

Falcon Arms

With this motion, any shoulder pain will vanish. Extend your arms to the sides. Next, cross one arm over the other at shoulder height in front of you. Bend your arms at the elbows and twist them so the palms are touching. Repeat with the opposing arm on top after releasing the hold after five breaths.

Neck Stretches with Assistance

Just so you know, our necks are under a lot of stress. Take your right arm and extend it over your head till the palm of your hand touches your left ear. Hold five breaths while you let your head rest on your right shoulder. On the other side, repeat.

Warrior I

This position can be modified for chair yoga, and you can still get shoulder-strengthening advantages without standing up and balancing. The regular variation of this pose requires you to stand up and engage your quads, glutes, and hamstrings to drop into a lunge. Furthermore, you'll stretch your hip flexors.

Face right and lean sideways on the chair so that the back of the seat is against the right side of the body. Set your right foot down on the floor. Your front foot should be parallel to the chair seat as you slowly stretch your left leg off the seat and swing it back behind you. As you breathe, contract your abs to raise your arms overhead and bring your hands together.

Knee to Ankle

One of the main stress points is the hip region. Sit up straight, bend your right knee and cross your right ankle over your left knee to ease the tension. Lean forward to stretch more deeply. After holding for five breaths, switch to the other side and repeat.

With a Twist, a Goddess

Open your legs wide and extend your toes for another excellent hip stretch. Reaching toward the floor, enclose your right arm inside your right leg. Your left arm should be raised to the ceiling, and your left palm should be in view. After holding for five breaths, switch to the other side and repeat.

Warriors II

Gain self-assurance while also stretching your entire body with this exercise. Tall and on the edge of your seat, sit. Your left leg should be extended behind you while you flex your right knee to the side and apply pressure through your outer heel. After holding for five breaths, switch to the other side and repeat.

Fold Forward

First, take a tall, straight seat. Next, cross your legs and allow your body, including your head and neck, to hang limp. Hold for however long you desire before rising to a sitting posture.

Chair Mountain Pose

One of the fundamental grounding postures in yoga, the mountain pose, is usually employed as a transitional or resting pose between other poses. By sitting on your yoga chair instead of standing, you can modify it for chair yoga. You'll continue to contract your abs, work on your posture, and focus on your breathing.

Your sit bones should be on the edge of the chair, your knees should be 90 degrees apart from your ankles, and your feet should be flat on the floor with your toes pointing forward. Your thighs ought to be hip-width apart and parallel.

Sit tall with your shoulders back, chest up, and eyes forward. As you inhale, picture a string falling from the top of your head, pulling you upward and stretching your spine. This will help you engage your core by drawing your belly button toward your spine and stretching your spine. Exhale, feeling anchored and linked to the chair as you sink into your sit bones. For 10 to 20 complete breaths, continue inhaling and exhaling in this manner.

Sitting Warrior

I'm from a Mounted Seated Pose while taking a deep breath and raising your arms above your head. Put your thumbs out and lace your fingers together. (It will appear as though you are "shooting" the ceiling.) Roll your shoulders back and exhale. Your shoulder capsule, made up of the helpful muscles that hold your shoulder joint together, will be in motion. Then, return your arms to your sides after five full breaths.

Bent Forward in a Chair

Inhale while placing your palms on your thighs. Exhale as you bend forward as comfortably as possible while maintaining a straight spine. Allowing the arms to dangle gently toward the floor will increase the stretch. Take five breaths minimum. As you turn back to your upright position, breathe in.

Chair "Uttanasana"

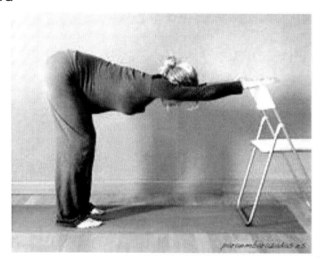

Lean forward keeping your back straight as your hands touch the back of the chair. Your head must be parallel to the back and remember to bend your knees slightly. This exercise helps to relax the leg muscles and abdomen.

Seated Twist

Raise your arms straight up, and your fingers pointed upward. Maintain a straight spine. After exhaling, turn to the right slowly. As you drop your arms, move your entire torso rather than your back. Place your right arm on the back of the chair very lightly. Look over your right shoulder and hold your position for five breaths. Repeat on the left side while returning to your starting position.

Safety advice: Resist the urge to tug on your chair and force the spin. This might result in severe pain or harm.

Eagle Arms Chair

Stretch your arms out by your sides and take a deep breath. Bring both your arms in front of you as you exhale. Swing your right arm under your left. With opposing hands, grab your shoulders. In essence, give yourself a big embrace. Breathe in and raise your elbows a little bit. Roll the shoulders back and down as you exhale and take a few breaths. On the opposite side, repeat. If you have good flexibility, consider releasing your hold on your shoulders and encircling your forearms in front of you while maintaining your elbows at chest level. Your left palm should hold your right hand's fingers.

Backward Arm

Hold your breath while you extend both arms at your sides, palms facing down. As you exhale, move both shoulders forward. Swing your hands lightly behind your back. To add some resistance, clasp your hands together and pull softly. Don't let go of your hold, though. Repeat with the opposite arms after five long breaths.

Five-Pointed Star Sitting

Breathe deeply and spread your arms to either side. Don't tense up your spine. Your fingers and the top of your skull should expand. Legs should be extended as straight as possible. Your head and limbs should work together to make the star that you are. Pause for five breaths.

Chair Pigeon

If your hips and glutes are tight, this chair yoga position is beneficial. With your core active, sit up straight. Raise and bend your right leg so your ankle lies on top of your left thigh, with your right knee on the side and your right shin aligned to the front edge of your chair's seat. You can bend at the hips to strengthen the pose and turn it into a forward bend.

Forward-Bent Chair Pose

Depending on your flexibility, this pose can stretch your hamstrings, low back, and shoulders. Exhale and hinge at the hips from the seated mountain pose to bend forward over your legs. Allowing your head to drop into your lap, extend your hands to rest on the floor or your ankles, depending on where you feel a healthy stretch. After taking a breath, rise to a sitting position and raise your arms aloft. For ten breaths, alternate between the forward fold and the upright sitting position.

Chair Extended Side Angle Pose

This pose can strengthen your obliques, shoulders, abs, and back while mobilizing your spine, enhancing posture and core strength. Start in the Seated Forward Fold but move your left hand's fingertips to the outside of your left foot instead. If you can't reach the floor, use a block. As you take a breath, turn your torso to the right. Open your chest as you raise your right arm and look up toward the ceiling. Hold for several deep breaths. On an out-breath, lower your back into the Forward Fold when ready.

CHAPTER 4: CHAIR YOGA ROUTINE EXERCISE TO SLEEP BETTER

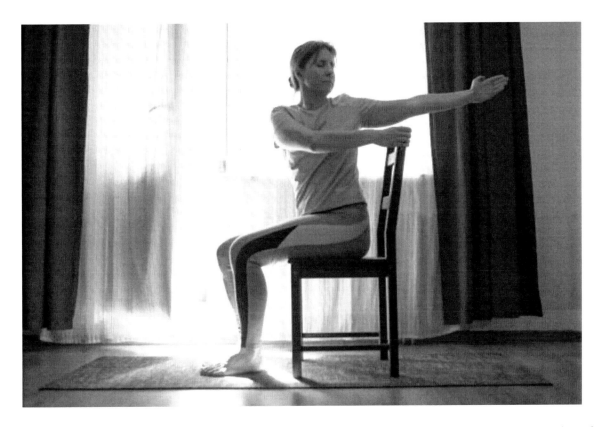

After a long day, deep breathing can aid in relaxation and winding down. Inhale deeply and steadily through both nostrils. Take many complete breaths, each lasting four counts (in and out). Then inhale for three counts and expel for six counts. Repeat several times. Increase the length of the exhalation as much as you can. Do only what is comfortable for you.

Practicing progressive relaxation in one of its many forms to relax the body. For instance, begin by focusing on your feet while taking deep, even breaths in and out. Focus on relaxing your feet, ankles, heels, calves, etc., with each exhalation. Some people find it relaxing to tense their muscles before letting them relax during an exhalation. As you relax, feel the tension leave the body part you are focusing on. Continue to relax every muscle in your body as you exhale. As you inhale and exhale, you can also focus on your breath or imagine a special word and repeat it yourself. Imagine yourself at a favorite spot and travel there.

Spend a moment unwinding before going to bed, it may be helpful to practice various chair yoga poses. Legs up the wall or on a chair (laying on the floor with your legs resting on a chair), seated forward bend, and sitting in an easy position with your legs crossed and your back against a wall are a few examples. Use these exercises you've learned to create a routine to be effective for you.

CONCLUSION

Exercise is a must for every age, but after a certain point, it becomes more of a necessity than an option to stay healthy and fit.

First and foremost, exercise has health advantages like stress reduction, weight loss, and bone mass restoration. It can lower your risk of developing chronic conditions like high blood pressure, stroke, and diabetes and enhance your general emotional and mental health. It also has been demonstrated that regular exercise enhances older persons' sleep quality.

A regular exercise regimen can lower your risk of falling by enhancing balance and coordination. Regular exercise increases muscle mass by causing minute tears in the muscle fibers that, when repaired, make the fibers stronger and larger.

With this 7-in-1 workout guide for seniors, you can kick-start your healthy routine anywhere and anytime. Just make sure to prepare your mind and body for this change. Set a schedule, stay hydrated, and eat healthy to stay strong.

Made in United States
North Haven, CT
16 March 2023

34157628R00111